Reconstructive Microsurgery:
Challenges and New Perspectives

Reconstructive Microsurgery: Challenges and New Perspectives

Editor

Albert H. Chao

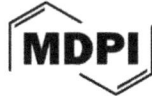 Basel • Beijing • Wuhan • Barcelona • Belgrade • Novi Sad • Cluj • Manchester

Editor
Albert H. Chao
Department of Plastic and
Reconstructive Surgery
Ohio State University
Columbus
USA

Editorial Office
MDPI
St. Alban-Anlage 66
4052 Basel, Switzerland

This is a reprint of articles from the Special Issue published online in the open access journal *Journal of Clinical Medicine* (ISSN 2077-0383) (available at: https://www.mdpi.com/journal/jcm/special_issues/H2548Q8N59).

For citation purposes, cite each article independently as indicated on the article page online and as indicated below:

Lastname, A.A.; Lastname, B.B. Article Title. *Journal Name* **Year**, *Volume Number*, Page Range.

ISBN 978-3-7258-1455-8 (Hbk)
ISBN 978-3-7258-1456-5 (PDF)
doi.org/10.3390/books978-3-7258-1456-5

© 2024 by the authors. Articles in this book are Open Access and distributed under the Creative Commons Attribution (CC BY) license. The book as a whole is distributed by MDPI under the terms and conditions of the Creative Commons Attribution-NonCommercial-NoDerivs (CC BY-NC-ND) license.

Contents

Dominika Lech, Jeremi Matysek, Robert Maksymowicz, Cyprian Strączek, Robert Marguła, Łukasz Krakowczyk, et al.
Maxillofacial Microvascular Free-Flap Reconstructions in Pediatric and Young Adult Patients—Outcomes and Potential Factors Influencing Success Rate
Reprinted from: *J. Clin. Med.* **2024**, *13*, 2015, doi:10.3390/jcm13072015 1

Z-Hye Lee, Ana Canzi, Jessie Yu and Edward I. Chang
Expanding the Armamentarium of Donor Sites in Microvascular Head and Neck Reconstruction
Reprinted from: *J. Clin. Med.* **2024**, *13*, 1311, doi:10.3390/jcm13051311 13

Min-Jeong Cho, Christopher A. Slater, Roman J. Skoracki and Albert H. Chao
Building Complex Autologous Breast Reconstruction Program: A Preliminary Experience
Reprinted from: *J. Clin. Med.* **2023**, *12*, 6810, doi:10.3390/jcm12216810 27

Yoon Jae Lee, Junnyeon Kim, Chae Rim Lee, Jun Hyeok Kim, Deuk Young Oh, Young Joon Jun and Suk-Ho Moon
Anterolateral Thigh Chimeric Flap: An Alternative Reconstructive Option to Free Flaps for Large Soft Tissue Defects
Reprinted from: *J. Clin. Med.* **2023**, *12*, 6723, doi:10.3390/jcm12216723 42

Brian Chuong, Kristopher Katira, Taylor Ramsay, John LoGiudice and Antony Martin
Reliability of Long Vein Grafts for Reconstruction of Massive Wounds
Reprinted from: *J. Clin. Med.* **2023**, *12*, 6209, doi:10.3390/jcm12196209 51

Johannes G. Schuderer, Huong T. Dinh, Steffen Spoerl, Jürgen Taxis, Mathias Fiedler, Josef M. Gottsauner, et al.
Risk Factors for Flap Loss: Analysis of Donor and Recipient Vessel Morphology in Patients Undergoing Microvascular Head and Neck Reconstructions
Reprinted from: *J. Clin. Med.* **2023**, *12*, 5206, doi:10.3390/jcm12165206 62

Nikita Roy, Christopher J. Alessandro, Taylor J. Ibelli, Arya A. Akhavan, Jake M. Sharaf, David Rabinovitch, et al.
The Expanding Utility of Robotic-Assisted Flap Harvest in Autologous Breast Reconstruction: A Systematic Review
Reprinted from: *J. Clin. Med.* **2023**, *12*, 4951, doi:10.3390/jcm12154951 74

Rihards P. Rocans, Janis Zarins, Evita Bine, Renars Deksnis, Margarita Citovica, Simona Donina and Biruta Mamaja
The Controlling Nutritional Status (CONUT) Score for Prediction of Microvascular Flap Complications in Reconstructive Surgery
Reprinted from: *J. Clin. Med.* **2023**, *12*, 4794, doi:10.3390/jcm12144794 88

Hyung-suk Yi, Byeong-seok Kim, Yoon-soo Kim, Jin-hyung Park and Hong-il Kim
What Is the Minimum Number of Sutures for Microvascular Anastomosis during Replantation?
Reprinted from: *J. Clin. Med.* **2023**, *12*, 2891, doi:10.3390/jcm12082891 99

Krzysztof Dowgierd, Rafał Pokrowiecki, Andrzej Myśliwiec and Łukasz Krakowczyk
Use of a Fibula Free Flap for Mandibular Reconstruction in Severe Craniofacial Microsomia in Children with Obstructive Sleep Apnea
Reprinted from: *J. Clin. Med.* **2023**, *12*, 1124, doi:10.3390/jcm12031124 109

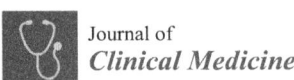 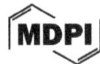

Article

Maxillofacial Microvascular Free-Flap Reconstructions in Pediatric and Young Adult Patients—Outcomes and Potential Factors Influencing Success Rate

Dominika Lech [1], Jeremi Matysek [1], Robert Maksymowicz [1], Cyprian Strączek [1], Robert Marguła [1], Łukasz Krakowczyk [2], Marcin Kozakiewicz [3] and Krzysztof Dowgierd [1,*]

[1] Department of Clinical Pediatrics, Head and Neck Surgery Clinic for Children and Young Adults, University of Warmia and Mazury, Żołnierska 18a Street, 10-561 Olsztyn, Poland; dominika.lech@student.uwm.edu.pl (D.L.); jeremi.matysek@student.uwm.edu.pl (J.M.); robert.maksymowicz@student.uwm.edu.pl (R.M.); cyprian.straczek@student.uwm.edu.pl (C.S.); robert.margula@student.uwm.edu.pl (R.M.)

[2] Oncological and Reconstructive Surgery Clinic, Branch of National Oncological Institute in Gliwice, Maria Sklodowska-Curie Institute—Oncology Centre (MSCI), Ul. Wybrzeże Armii Krajowej 15, 44-100 Gliwice, Poland

[3] Department of Maxillofacial Surgery, Medical Univeristy of Lodz, 113 Żeromskiego Str., 90-549 Lodz, Poland; marcin.kozakiewicz@umed.lodz.pl

* Correspondence: krzysztofdowgierd@gmail.com

Abstract: Background: Maxillofacial microvascular free-flap reconstructions are significant interventions in the management of congenital defects, traumatic injuries, malignancies, and iatrogenic complications in pediatric and young adult patients. Craniofacial disorders within this demographic can result in profound functional, cosmetic, and psychosocial impairments, highlighting the critical need for thorough investigation into factors that may influence procedural success and postoperative quality of life. This retrospective chart review aims to examine the outcomes and potential influencing factors, aiming to offer valuable insights into optimizing the effectiveness of these reconstructions and improving patient outcomes. **Methods**: A single head and neck surgical team performed all the included 136 procedures. Demographic and surgical patient data were recorded. Type of transfer performed in each recipient site and major complications were analyzed. Relevant influencing factors, such as age, gender, and etiology of defect were determined using the ANOVA test and χ^2 test of independence. **Results**: The results indicate a 90% success rate. No significant relationship was found between the incidence of total flap loss and patient age, etiology, or graft source. The maxillary reconstructions showed a higher incidence of total flap loss compared to mandibular reconstructions (11 vs. 3 cases). **Conclusions**: Despite the high success rate, the findings underline the necessity for further research to validate these observations and enhance surgical methods for pediatric and young adult patients.

Keywords: pediatric; free flap; microvascular reconstruction; head and neck; outcomes; success rate; complications

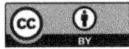

1. Introduction

Head and neck disorders in pediatric and young adult patients can result in significant functional and cosmetic deformities [1], originating from causes such as congenital defects, traumatic injuries, malignancies, and iatrogenic complications. Microvascular free-flap reconstructions have become essential in addressing these complex deformations, transforming the field of head and neck reconstruction by enabling the transfer of reliable bone and soft tissue from distant sites using microsurgical techniques [2]. In the context of pediatric and young adult patients, however, there exists a significant gap in detailed research explaining the specific impacts and nuances of these procedures [1,3–5]. While previous studies have explored potential determinants influencing the success rates of microvascular free-flap reconstructions [1,3,6,7], a consensus regarding these factors remains unclear, indicating the need for further investigation.

The physiological and developmental characteristics unique to youth require specialized approaches different from those used in adult populations [8]. By examining variables such as age, sex, etiology of the maxillofacial defect, graft source, and recipient site location, this research seeks to understand the relationship between these factors and surgical outcomes. Through a detailed analysis of a cohort comprising 136 pediatric and young adult patients who underwent maxillofacial microvascular free-flap reconstructions, this study aims to identify key determinants impacting surgical success. The findings are expected to provide a basis for future research aimed at improving the effectiveness and enhancing the post-surgical quality of life for pediatric and young adult patients undergoing these procedures [9].

2. Materials and Methods

This is a retrospective chart review from August 2011 to June 2023. Data were collected from the Maxillofacial Surgery for Children and Young Adults Division in the Head and Neck Clinic, Regional Specialized Children's Hospital in Olsztyn, Poland. This study included patients from 1 to 25 years of age. A total of 136 procedures performed on 136 patients with complete medical records were analyzed. Patients were categorized by recipient site anatomical location, and major complications were recorded.

2.1. Procedures and Techniques

The free-flap auto-transplantation procedure began with the resection of pathology, resulting in tissue loss in the recipient site. Next, the flap was harvested from the donor site but remained connected to surrounding tissue by at least one artery and one vein. Simultaneously, the recipient site was surgically dissected to prepare the recipient artery, the facial artery, and vein, predominantly the facial vein, for anastomosis with the vascular pedicle of the free flap. The free flap was brought to the defect area and the vessels of the flap were anastomosed with the vessels of the recipient site, under the control of a microscope. After reconnection, the free flap was sutured to the defect, while the medical team monitored blood flow in the anastomosed vessels to ensure patency. Meanwhile, the donor site was primarily closed.

2.2. Terms

Iatrogenic etiology refers to cases where surgical interventions, initially intended to address a medical condition or trauma, inadvertently result in further complications or damage requiring microvascular free-flap reconstructive surgical intervention.

Lower limb nerve flap refers to a vascularized free flap containing skin, subcutaneous tissue with or without muscles and sural or tibial nerves acquired from the lower limb.

2.3. Data Collection and Statistical Analysis

Data for this study were extracted from electronic health records. A database was established for analysis. Recorded parameters included gender, age, etiology of the condition, recipient and donor sites, as well as postoperative complications.

The statistical analysis was performed using STATGRAPHICS Centurion 19 (StatPoint, Tulsa, OK, USA). The ANOVA test was utilized to determine relationships between age as a continuous variable and recipient site complications, etiology, and total flap loss. The χ^2 test of independence was applied to assess relationships among categorical variables, including age groups, gender, recipient site complications, donor site, etiology, and the incidence of total flap loss. Age groups were categorized as follows: less than 5 years, 5 to 10 years, 11 to 15 years, 16 to 20 years, and over 20 years. A threshold of $p < 0.05$ was set to determine statistical significance.

3. Results

This study included 136 young patients who underwent microvascular free-flap reconstructions, comprising 76 females and 60 males. The median age was 14 years, ranging from 1 to 25 years. Table 1 accurately delineates the demographic and clinical data, illustrating gender distribution, etiology, recipient and donor sites, and recipient site complications. The predominant etiology of the underlying pathology was neoplastic in nature, accounting for 82 out of 136 cases (60.3%), followed by congenital defects in 39 cases (28.7%). The most frequently reconstructed sites were the maxilla (56 out of 136 cases, 41.2%) and mandible (55 out of 136 cases, 40.4%). The fibula (47 out of 136 cases, 34.6%) and iliac crest (44 out of 136 cases, 32.4%) were the most harvested flaps. Out of the 136 procedures performed, 122 resulted in successful free-flap survival, while 14 cases experienced total flap loss, yielding an overall success rate of 89.7%. Postoperative complications included total flap necrosis in 14 cases (10.3%), partial flap necrosis in 11 cases (8.1%), abscess formation in 4 cases (2.9%), and nerve palsy in 1 case (0.7%). The distribution of total flap necrosis was 11 in maxillary reconstructions and 3 in mandibular reconstructions. Within the maxillary reconstruction group, the total flap loss was distributed among donor sites as follows: five cases from the iliac crest (representing 20.8% of all iliac crest flaps transplanted to the maxilla), five from the fibula (35.7% of all fibular flaps to the maxilla), and one from the medial condyle of the femur (constituting 7% of all such flaps to the maxilla). Within the mandibular reconstruction group, the total flap loss was distributed among donor sites as follows: two cases from the fibula (6.1% of all fibular flaps to the mandible) and one case from the iliac crest (representing 5% of all such flaps to the mandible).

Table 1. Demographics.

	Frequency	Percent
Sex		
Female	76	55.9%
Male	60	44.1%
Etiology		
Congenital	39	28.7%
Oncological	82	60.3%
Traumatic	5	3.7%
Iatrogenic	10	7.4%
Recipient Site		
Mandible	55	40.4%
Maxilla	56	41.2%
Soft tissue	17	12.5%
Orbit	4	2.9%
Facial nerve	4	2.9%
Donor Site		
Iliac crest	44	32.4%
Medial condyle of femur	15	11.0%
Fibula	47	34.6%
Antero-lateral thigh	17	12.5%
Forearm	7	5.1%
Gracilis muscle	4	2.9%
Lower limb nerve	2	1.5%
Recipient Site Complications		
Nerve palsy	1	0.7%
Abscess	4	2.9%
Partial flap necrosis	11	8.1%
Total flap necrosis	14	10.3%
None	106	78%
Total	136	100%

3.1. Patient's Age at the Time of Surgery and Total Flap Loss

Table 2 shows that the mean age at the time of microsurgical reconstruction was 13.5 (±4.98), with a median of 14 years. For patients who had a successful procedure, the mean age was 13.4 (±5.0), with a median of 14 years. In contrast, the mean age for those with flap failure was 14.2 (±4.95), with a median of 14.5 years. Statistical analysis indicated no significant age difference between the patients with flap survival and those with flap loss [F (4,131) = 0.33, p = 0.57], which is presented in Figure 1.

Table 2. Summary statistics of patient's age by flap survival or total flap loss.

	Count	Average	Median	Standard Deviation	Minimum	Maximum
Flap survived	122	13.4	14.0	5.0	1.0	25.0
Total Flap Loss	14	14.2	14.5	4.95	4.0	22.0
Total	136	13.5	14.0	4.98	1.0	25.0

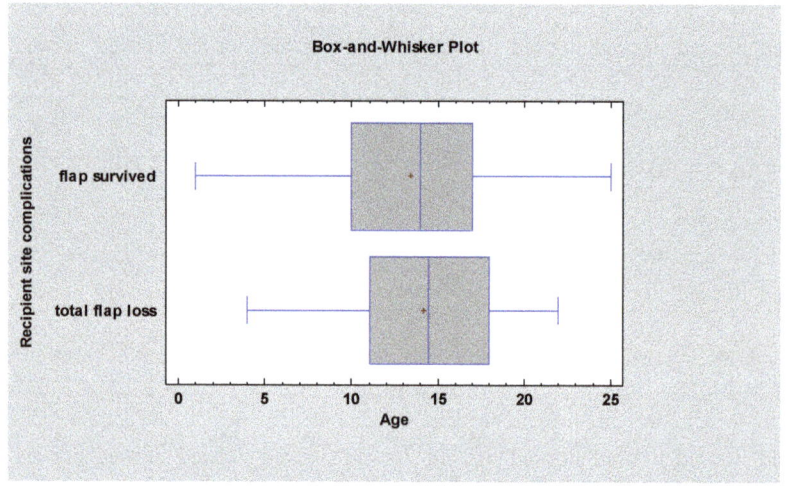

Figure 1. There is no age-dependent relationship of total flap loss.

3.2. Gender, Etiology of the Underlying Pathology, and the Occurrence of Total Flap Loss

Figure 2 provides an overview of the data. In evaluating the impact of etiology on the incidence of total flap loss and flap survival, the oncological group demonstrated a total flap loss in eight cases, which constituted 5.88% of all one hundred and thirty-six cases. The congenital etiologies had a lower incidence of total flap loss, with six cases representing 4.41% of all reconstructions performed. Both trauma and iatrogenic categories maintained a 100% flap survival rate with no instances of total flap loss. Statistical analysis revealed no significant differences in the incidence of total flap loss across etiology groups [χ^2 (3, N = 136) = 2.84, p = 0.42].

Table 3 indicates that female patients underwent more flap transfers than male patients (n = 76 vs. n = 60) and experienced a higher incidence of total flap loss (n = 11 vs. n = 3). As a result, the success rate was lower among females (86%) than males (95%). However, statistical analysis did not reveal any significant differences between the genders in terms of flap survivability [χ^2 (1, N = 136) = 3.26, p = 0.07].

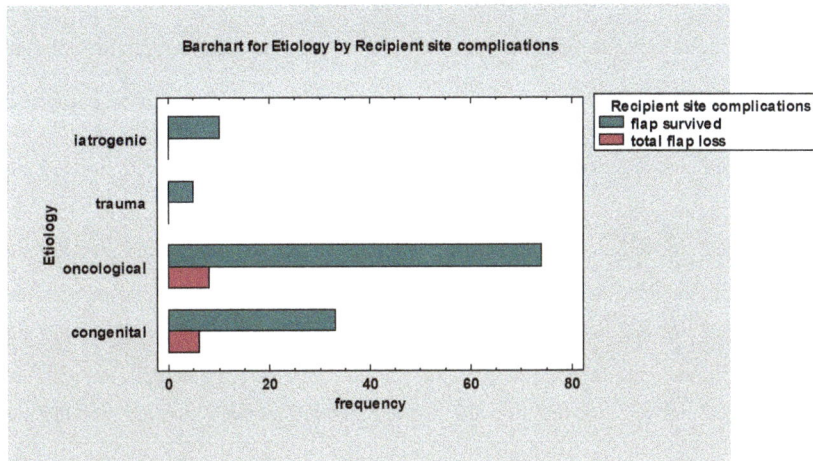

Figure 2. Numbers of total flap losses and flap survival by etiology of reconstruction.

Table 3. Summary of number of procedures resulting in flap survival or total flap loss with calculated success rate by gender.

Gender	Number of Procedures with Flap Survival	Number of Procedures with Total Flap Loss	Total Number of Procedures	Success Rate
Female	65	11	76	85.5%
Male	57	3	60	95%

3.3. Age and the Occurrence of Recipient Site Complications

Figure 3 provides an overview of the data. No recipient site complications were recorded in 106 procedures. The mean age of patients without recipient site complications was 13.26 (±5.11) with a median age of 14 years. The most common complication in recipient site was total flap loss ($n = 14$) with a mean age at the time of procedure of 14.21 (±4.95) and a median age of 14.5 years. Eleven procedures resulted in partial flap loss with a mean age of 14.55 (±3.56) and patients' median age of 15 years. The recipient site complication was abscess in four procedures, with a mean and median age at the time of surgery of 14.00 (±6.78) and 14.5 years, respectively. One procedure resulted in nerve palsy in a 14 y.o. patient. No significant relationship was found between age and recipient site complications [$F (4, 131) = 0.26, p = 0.90$].

3.4. Occurrence of Recipient Site Complications between Age Groups and Age Group Specific Success Rate

Table 4 provides a summary of recipient site complications categorized by age groups. The 16 to 20-year-old group had the highest incidence of recipient site complications, which also correlated with having the highest number of procedures and the highest number of cases resulting in total flap loss. The fewest complications were noted in patients under 5 years of age, with this group having only one case of total flap loss and no other documented complications. The group aged 6 to 10 years demonstrated the highest success rate at 92%. Statistical analysis revealed no significant differences in the incidence of recipient site complications across age groups [$\chi^2 (16, N = 136) = 7.94, p = 0.95$]. Additionally, Figure 4 indicated that there was no significant relationship between age groups and the number of total flap losses [$\chi^2 (4, N = 136) = 0.24, p = 0.99$].

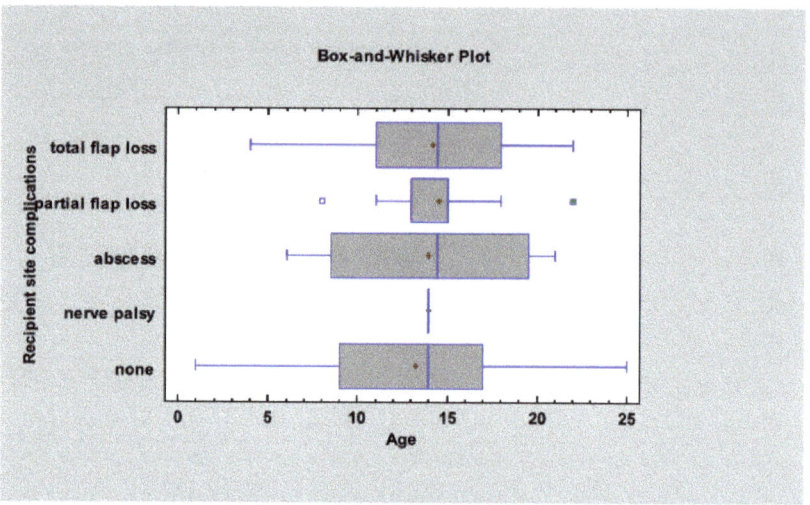

Figure 3. There is no age-dependent relationship of recipient site complications.

Table 4. Summary of occurrence of recipient site complications by age group with calculated success rate for each age group.

Age Group	Number of Complications		Total Number of Procedures	Success Rate	Complication Rate
	Other	Total Flap Loss			
Less than 5 y.o.	0	1	8	87.5%	0%
6 to 10 y.o.	2	2	25	92%	8%
11 to 15 y.o.	6	4	39	89.7%	15.4%
16 to 20 y.o.	6	6	56	89.3%	10.7%
Greater than 20 y.o.	2	1	8	87.5%	25%

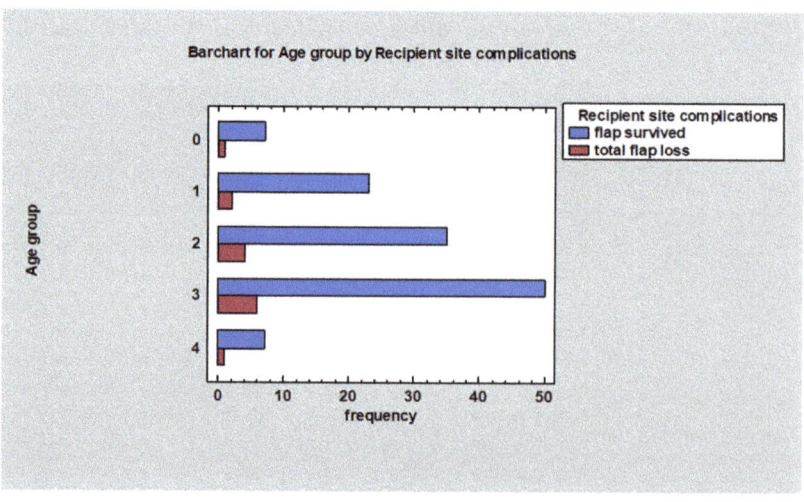

Figure 4. Number of procedures resulting in flap survival or total flap loss for age groups. Numbers on Y axis are labels of age groups ("0"= less than 5 y.o.; "1"= 6 to 10 y.o.; "2" = 11 to 15 y.o.; "3" = 16 to 20 y.o.; "4" = greater than 20 y.o.).

3.5. Recipient Site, Recipient Site Complication and Flap Survival

Table 5 highlights a significant discrepancy in the incidence of total flap loss between the maxilla and mandible groups. The maxilla group, with the highest number of transplants ($n = 56$), also had the highest incidence of total flap loss ($n = 11$), resulting in a success rate of 80.4% for free-flap transplants in this group. In contrast, of the 55 free-flap transplantations to the mandible, only 3 resulted in total flap loss, yielding a success rate of 94.6% for mandibular reconstructions. The difference in total flap loss between the two sites was statistically significant ($p < 0.05$) [χ^2 (4, $N = 136$) = 9.56, $p = 0.049$]. For the maxillary transplants, 24 (42.9%) flaps were harvested from the iliac crest, 14 (25%) from the fibula, 14 (25%) from the medial condyle of the femur, 3 (5.4%) from the anterolateral thigh, and 1 from the forearm. In the 55 mandibular transplants, there were 33 fibula flaps (60%), 20 (36.4%) flaps from the iliac crest and 2 (3.6%) flaps from the medical condyle of femur. In the groups undergoing soft tissue, orbital, and facial nerve microsurgical reconstruction, there were no instances of total flap loss, leading to success rates of 100% in these categories.

Table 5. Summary of numbers of complications in recipient site with calculated success rate for each recipient site.

Recipient Site	Number of Flap Survival	Number of Total Flap Loss	Total Number of Procedures	Success Rate
Maxilla	45	11	56	80.4%
Mandible	52	3	55	94.6%
Soft tissue	17	0	17	100%
Orbit	4	0	4	100%
Facial nerve	4	0	4	100%

Table 6 indicates that the maxilla group experienced the highest number of recipient site complications, followed by the mandible and soft tissue groups. There were no reported complications for free-flap transfers to the orbital or facial nerve. Excluding total flap loss, the complication rate for free-flap transfers to the maxilla was 10.7%, while transfers to the mandible had a complication rate of 16.4%. The results of the χ^2 test suggest no significant association between the recipient sites and the occurrence of complications [χ^2 (4, $N = 136$) = 7.10, $p = 0.13$].

Table 6. Summary of number of procedures with and without complications in recipient site.

Recipient Site	Number of Procedures with Complications (Including Total Flap Loss)	Number of Procedures without Complications	Total Number of Procedures
Maxilla	17	39	56
Mandible	12	43	55
Soft tissue	1	16	17
Orbit	0	4	4
Facial nerve	0	4	4

4. Discussion

This study conducted an extensive examination of maxillofacial microvascular free-flap reconstructions in a pediatric and young adult cohort, yielding significant insights into the success rates and factors influencing outcomes. The observed success rate of 89.71% in our study, while notable, is somewhat lower compared to the success rates typically reported in the existing literature, which often exceed 94% [1,3–5,9–12]. In a study by Liu et al. (2018) focusing on pediatric head and neck reconstruction, a higher success rate of 95.6% was reported [1]. However, it is essential to highlight the differences in the distribution of recipient sites between the two studies. Our research found the maxilla (55 out of 136 cases) and mandible (55 cases) to be the most common recipient sites, with the maxilla having the highest incidence of total flap loss. Notably, the success rate for mandibular reconstructions in our study was 94.55%, closely aligning with the higher success rates reported in the literature. In contrast, the study by Liu et al. primarily involved mandibular reconstructions (88 out of 135 cases), with only nine cases of maxillary reconstructions. Despite their conclusion of no significant relationship between recipient site and total flap loss, the predominance of mandibular reconstructions in their study, which aligns closely with the higher success rates in our mandibular cases, might partially explain the overall greater results observed in their findings.

In our analysis, we specifically examined the relationship between patient age and the incidence of total flap loss. It has been observed that children under ten years of age might be at a heightened risk of lower success rates in these procedures [1]. The potential underlying factors attributed to this finding include the reduced diameter of vasculature in younger patients, arterial vasospasms, and heightened complexity in performing surgical techniques on smaller anatomical structures. Regardless of these findings, our data did not demonstrate a significant relationship between patient age and the incidence of total flap loss. Interestingly, this result is consistent with another substantial study involving 102 patients, where a similar lack of relationship between age and surgical success in microvascular reconstructions was observed [13]. This parallel outcome in a separate large-scale study reinforces the notion that age, while an important consideration, may not be as critical a determinant of flap survival.

We investigated the potential relationship between patient gender and the incidence of total flap loss. Our examination revealed a borderline statistical significance ($p = 0.071$), suggesting a tentative yet not statistically validated trend towards a higher risk of total flap loss in female patients. However, given the marginal nature of this finding, it necessitates further investigation with an expanded pediatric sample size to establish a more definitive conclusion. The literature presents varied perspectives on the influence of gender in head and neck reconstructions. For example, Loupatatzi et al. identified female gender as one of the factors associated with increased complications in head and neck cancer reconstructions, alongside pre-operative radiation therapy and extended surgery duration [14]. In contrast, Rohleder et al. reported no significant gender-related differences in the postoperative outcomes of free-flap reconstructions in the head and neck region [15]. It is important to note, however, that these studies predominantly involved adult populations, with mean ages notably above the pediatric range, and thereby limiting the applicability of their findings to a younger demographic.

A striking finding was the higher incidence of total flap loss in maxillary reconstructions compared to mandibular ones. Specifically, the maxilla experienced 11 cases of total flap necrosis out of 55 reconstructions, translating to a success rate of 80.36%, markedly lower than the 94.55% rate observed for mandibular reconstructions. This contrast becomes even more pronounced when compared to adult maxillary reconstruction success rates, which typically hover around 95% in the literature [16,17]. However, it aligns more closely with recent findings in pediatric patients, such as those reported by Burns et al. (2023), who observed a 23% total flap loss in pediatric maxillary reconstructions [18].

The absence of any total flap loss instances in reconstructions involving soft tissues, orbital regions, and facial nerves is noteworthy. The results are consistent with the noted trend that flaps incorporating bone have a nearly five-fold higher failure rate compared to those consisting entirely of soft tissue. This is likely attributable to the fact that in bone defect reconstructions, the positioning of both the flap and its pedicle is dictated by the bony defect, offering limited flexibility for alteration [19].

Moreover, the findings of our study hold potential utility in empowering both patients and their parents to make more informed decisions regarding free-flap microvascular reconstruction. It is an ethical obligation for physicians to provide comprehensive information to patients, encompassing diagnosis, planned treatment, postoperative complications, and success rates. Agozzino et al.'s study has contributed valuable insights into patient satisfaction and the frequency of legal claims concerning surgical procedures. The research revealed that patients who received both written consent and oral information about procedures exhibited higher satisfaction with surgical treatment compared to those who received written consent alone. Remarkably, 19.6% of individuals receiving both written and oral information reported feeling influenced to varying degrees. Notably, information regarding postoperative complications and success rates received limited attention from physicians. However, when conveyed, such information correlated with increased satisfaction with treatment and reduced patient's anxiety [20]. These findings underscore the importance of effective communication, providing reliable data on postoperative complications and success rates in the context of free-flap microvascular reconstructions. This could potentially enhance the satisfaction of patients and their parents while concurrently reducing the incidence of legal claims. Nevertheless, the study is subject to certain limitations. Primarily, it was conducted in general surgery units in Italy, specifically on adult patients capable of legally consenting to surgery. Consequently, the generalizability of these findings to pediatric settings is restricted to patients' parents. Additionally, the study relied on face-to-face interviews conducted several days after patients had received written consent, introducing a potential risk of recall bias.

In our clinical practice, maxillofacial free-flap reconstructive surgeries are often necessitated by various etiologies, including oncological, traumatic, and congenital factors. These procedures not only address medical needs, such as tumor resections, but also significantly enhance craniofacial function, repair defects, and mitigate facial deformities. However, it is crucial to recognize that these surgeries invariably alter the patient's facial appearance, underscoring the importance of properly informing both patients and parents about this fact. Parental involvement in decision-making regarding pediatric reconstructive surgery is pivotal, as some advocate for proactive surgical intervention, while others suggest waiting until the child can actively participate in the decision-making process [21]. Incorporating intervention strategies, such as psychological support before and after surgery, as well as potential corrective cosmetic procedures, enables the effective management of their psychological burdens postoperatively and may help to tone down the negative psychosocial consequences. In particular, for appearance-sensitive adolescents, counseling pre- and postoperatively could be required to prepare them for the resultant changes. This aligns with findings from studies on head and neck reconstructions, which highlight the significant impact on patients' psychological well-being, especially among vulnerable groups such as women with a history of anxiety or depression [22,23]. Similarly, research on patients with tongue cancer undergoing resection procedures emphasizes the variations in quality of life and psychological status, with more extensive surgeries often resulting in worse outcomes [24]. Therefore, it is critical for healthcare professionals to advocate for patients considering surgery, facilitate informed decision-making, and mitigate emotional and social obstacles by openly discussing potential challenges pre-operatively, developing coping mechanisms, and educating parents and peers to reduce post-surgery psychological distress [21].

Despite advancements in reconstructive surgery, the management of complications following flap failure remains an area with significant gaps in understanding and exploration [25]. In our practice, the approach entails the removal of the necrotic tissue flap followed by reoperation. Additionally, thorough discussions with the patient and parents regarding the available options, potential risks, and expected outcomes are deemed essential. Identifying reversible causes for the initial flap failure is also emphasized to reduce risks in subsequent procedures. This approach requires a comprehensive assessment of the patient's medical status aimed at optimizing their candidacy for potential subsequent interventions, with a specific focus directed towards mitigating any underlying pathological factors implicated in the initial flap failure. Given supportive findings for the efficacy of a second free flap for salvage reconstruction, this approach is preferred whenever feasible. Nonetheless, it is crucial to consider individual patient circumstances, including comorbidities and recipient site characteristics. Ultimately, the objective is to achieve optimal outcomes encompassing cosmesis, function, and complication rates, recognizing the need for a tailored approach to maximize success rates in each case [25].

The retrospective design of this study necessitated the use of electronic medical records, which introduces the possibility of substantial data loss due to incomplete documentation from the healthcare providers or variations in medical terminology usage. Additionally, crucial information regarding free-flap dimensions and vasculature diameter was unavailable, potentially impacting the outcomes of free-flap microvascular reconstruction, including the risk of flap failure. The recommendations for further studies underscore the pressing need for standardization in both flap selection and perioperative care for pediatric patients undergoing free-flap microvascular reconstruction. Given the scarcity of studies in the literature in this area, it is imperative that future research prioritizes the development of protocols and guidelines aimed at standardizing the selection of appropriate flaps, surgical techniques, and postoperative care measures. By establishing standardized procedures, the potential for enhancing the overall success rate of these reconstructions and improving outcomes for pediatric patients becomes evident. Additionally, there is a critical need for further exploration into the harmonization of perioperative care, particularly in the realm of anesthetic management for pediatric patients undergoing such procedures. The perioperative period significantly influences complication rates and overall outcomes. Therefore, the implementation of standardized protocols for anesthesia, encompassing preoperative assessment, intraoperative monitoring, and postoperative pain management, is essential for mitigating postoperative complications effectively. Enhanced coordination and consistency in perioperative care have the potential to augment the success rate of reconstructions and contribute to better patient outcomes. Further scientific inquiry of a similar nature is warranted to validate and build upon our findings, ultimately advancing the field and improving patient care practices.

5. Conclusions

The aim of our study was to identify key factors influencing the success of maxillofacial microvascular free-flap reconstructions in pediatric and young adult patients. Our findings point towards the importance of the recipient site, particularly the challenges associated with maxillary reconstructions. The lack of significant correlation with age and gender shifts focus to site-specific variables rather than demographic ones. This study, therefore, underscores the need for specialized surgical strategies for maxillary reconstructions in the young population.

Author Contributions: Conceptualization, D.L., J.M., R.M. (Robert Maksymowicz), C.S. and K.D.; data curation, D.L., J.M., R.M. (Robert Maksymowicz), C.S. and M.K.; formal analysis, D.L., J.M., R.M. (Robert Maksymowicz), C.S., R.M. (Robert Marguła), Ł.K., M.K. and K.D.; funding acquisition, K.D.; investigation, D.L., J.M., R.M. (Robert Maksymowicz), and C.S.; methodology, D.L., J.M., R.M. (Robert Maksymowicz), C.S., R.M. (Robert Marguła), M.K. and K.D.; project administration, D.L. and K.D.; resources, Ł.K.; software, M.K.; supervision, Ł.K. and K.D.; Validation, D.L., J.M., R.M. (Robert Maksymowicz), C.S., R.M. (Robert Marguła), Ł.K., M.K. and K.D.; visualization, D.L., R.M. (Robert Maksymowicz), and M.K.; writing—original draft, D.L., J.M., R.M. (Robert Maksymowicz), C.S. and R.M. (Robert Marguła); writing—review and editing, D.L., J.M., R.M. (Robert Maksymowicz), C.S., R.M. (Robert Marguła), and K.D. All authors have read and agreed to the published version of the manuscript.

Funding: This research received no external funding.

Institutional Review Board Statement: The study was conducted in accordance with the Declaration of Helsinki, and approved by the Institutional Review Board (or Ethics Committee) of Regional Specialized Children's Hospital in Olsztyn, (5a ZE//2024/WSSD; 30 January 2024).

Informed Consent Statement: Informed consent was obtained from all subjects involved in the study.

Data Availability Statement: The data are available upon request from the corresponding author.

Conflicts of Interest: The authors declare no conflicts of interest.

References

1. Liu, S.; Zhang, W.-B.; Yu, Y.; Wang, Y.; Mao, C.; Guo, C.-B.; Yu, G.-Y.; Peng, X. Free Flap Transfer for Pediatric Head and Neck Reconstruction: What Factors Influence Flap Survival? *Laryngoscope* **2019**, *129*, 1915–1921. [CrossRef] [PubMed]
2. Patel, S.Y.; Kim, D.D.; Ghali, G.E. Maxillofacial Reconstruction Using Vascularized Fibula Free Flaps and Endosseous Implants. *Oral Maxillofac. Surg. Clin. North Am.* **2019**, *31*, 259–284. [CrossRef] [PubMed]
3. Upton, J.; Guo, L. Pediatric free tissue transfer: A 29-year experience with 433 transfers. *Plast Reconstr. Surg.* **2008**, *121*, 1725–1737. [CrossRef] [PubMed]
4. Bilkay, U.; Tiftikcioglu, Y.O.; Temiz, G.; Ozek, C.; Akin, Y. Free-tissue transfers for reconstruction of oromandibular area in children. *Microsurgery* **2008**, *28*, 91–98. [CrossRef] [PubMed]
5. Markiewicz, M.R.; Ruiz, R.L.; Pirgousis, P.; Bryan Bell, R.; Dierks, E.J.; Edwards, S.P.; Fernandes, R. Microvascular Free Tissue Transfer for Head and Neck Reconstruction in Children. *J. Craniofacial Surg.* **2016**, *27*, 846–856. [CrossRef] [PubMed]
6. James, J.; Seyidova, N.; Takyi, E.; Oleru, O.; Taub, P.J. Microvascular Soft Tissue Reconstruction Outcomes and Risk Factors in Pediatric Patients Undergoing Head and Neck Reconstruction. *FACE* **2024**, *5*, 26–33. [CrossRef]
7. Sun, Z.Y.; Chen, Y.M.; Xie, L.; Yang, X.; Ji, T. Free flap reconstruction in paediatric patients with head and neck cancer: Clinical considerations for comprehensive care. *Int. J. Oral Maxillofac. Surg.* **2020**, *49*, 1416–1420. [CrossRef] [PubMed]
8. Weizman, N.; Gil, Z.; Wasserzug, O.; Amir, A.; Gur, E.; Margalit, N.; Fliss, D.M. Surgical ablation and free flap reconstruction in children with malignant head and neck tumors. *Skull Base* **2011**, *21*, 165–170. [CrossRef] [PubMed]
9. Alkureishi, L.W.T.; Purnell, C.A.; Park, P.; Bauer, B.S.; Fine, N.A.; Sisco, M. Long-term Outcomes After Pediatric Free Flap Reconstruction. *Ann. Plast Surg.* **2018**, *81*, 449–455. [CrossRef]
10. Crosby, M.A.; Martin, J.W.; Robb, G.L.; Chang, D.W. Pediatric mandibular recon- struction using a vascularized fibula flap. *Head Neck J. Sci. Spec.* **2008**, *30*, 311–319. [CrossRef] [PubMed]
11. Warren, S.M.; Borud, L.J.; Brecht, L.E.; Longaker, M.T.; Siebert, J.W. Microvascular reconstruction of the pediatric mandible. *Plast. Reconstr. Surg.* **2007**, *119*, 649–661. [CrossRef] [PubMed]
12. Wolf, R.; Ringel, B.; Zissman, S.; Shapira, U.; Duek, I.; Muhanna, N.; Horowitz, G.; Zaretski, A.; Yanko, R.; Derowe, A.; et al. Free flap transfers for head and neck and skull base reconstruction in children and adolescents—Early and late outcomes. *Int. J. Pediatr. Otorhinolaryngol.* **2020**, *138*, 110299. [CrossRef] [PubMed]
13. Starnes-Roubaud, M.J.; Hanasono, M.M.; Kupferman, M.E.; Liu, J.; Chang, E.I. Microsurgical reconstruction following oncologic resection in pediatric patients: A 15-year experience. *Ann. Surg. Oncol.* **2017**, *24*, 4009–4016. [CrossRef] [PubMed]
14. Loupatatzi, A.; Stavrianos, S.; Karantonis, F.F.; Machairas, A.; Rapidis, A.D.; Kokkalis, G.; Papadopoulos, O. Are Females Predisposed to Complications in Head and Neck Cancer Free Flap Reconstruction? *J. Oral Maxillofac. Surg.* **2014**, *72*, 178–185. [CrossRef] [PubMed]
15. Rohleder, N.H.; Heimüller, S.; Wolff, K.D.; Kesting, M.R. Influence of biological sex on intra- and postoperative course of microvascular free flap reconstructive surgery in the head and neck region: A retrospective analysis involving 215 patients. *Adv. Oral Maxillofac. Surg.* **2022**, *7*, 100307. [CrossRef]
16. Costa, H.; Zenha, H.; Sequeira, H.; Coelho, G.; Gomes, N.; Pinto, C.; Martins, J.; Santos, D.; Andresen, C. Microsurgical reconstruction of the maxilla: Algorithm and concepts. *J. Plast. Reconstr. Aesthetic Surg.* **2015**, *68*, e89–e104. [CrossRef] [PubMed]
17. Mücke, T.; Hölzle, F.; Loeffelbein, D.J.; Ljubic, A.; Kesting, M.; Wolff, K.-D.; Mitchell, D.A. Maxillary reconstruction using microvascular free flaps. *Oral Surg. Oral Med. Oral Pathol. Oral Radiol. Endodontology* **2011**, *111*, 51–57. [CrossRef] [PubMed]
18. Burns, H.R.; Yim, N.H.; Hashemi, A.S.A.; Upadhyaya, R.M.; Montgomery, A.; Dimachkieh, A.L.; Pederson, W.C.; Buchanan, E.P. Pediatric Maxilla-Mandible Oncoplastic Reconstruction: A 25 Patient Case Series. *FACE* **2023**, *4*, 495–504. [CrossRef]
19. Kroll, S.S.; Schusterman, M.A.; Reece, G.P.; Miller, M.J.; Evans, G.R.; Robb, G.L.; Baldwin, B.J. Choice of flap and incidence of free flap success. *Plast. Reconstr Surg.* **1996**, *98*, 459–463. [CrossRef] [PubMed]
20. Agozzino, E.; Borrelli, S.; Cancellieri, M.; Carfora, F.M.; Di Lorenzo, T.; Attena, F. Does written informed consent adequately inform surgical patients? A cross sectional study. *BMC Med. Ethics* **2019**, *20*, 1. [CrossRef] [PubMed]
21. Bemmels, H.; Biesecker, B.; Schmidt, J.L.; Krokosky, A.; Guidotti, R.; Sutton, E.J. Psychological and social factors in undergoing reconstructive surgery among individuals with craniofacial conditions: An exploratory study. *Cleft Palate Craniofac. J.* **2013**, *50*, 158–167. [CrossRef] [PubMed]
22. Zebolsky, A.L.; Ochoa, E.; Badran, K.W.; Heaton, C.; Park, A.; Seth, R.; Knott, P.D. Appearance-Related Distress and Social Functioning after Head and Neck Microvascular Reconstruction. *Laryngoscope* **2021**, *131*, E2204–E2211. [CrossRef] [PubMed]
23. Zebolsky, A.L.; Patel, N.; Heaton, C.M.; Park, A.M.; Seth, R.; Knott, P.D. Patient-Reported Aesthetic and Psychosocial Outcomes After Microvascular Reconstruction for Head and Neck Cancer. *JAMA Otolaryngol. Head Neck Surg.* **2021**, *147*, 1035–1044. [CrossRef] [PubMed]

24. Suzuki, K.; Nishio, N.; Kimura, H.; Tokura, T.; Kishi, S.; Ozaki, N.; Fujimoto, Y.; Sone, M. Comparison of quality of life and psychological distress in patients with tongue cancer undergoing a total/subtotal glossectomy or extended hemiglossectomy and free flap transfer: A prospective evaluation. *Int. J. Oral Maxillofac. Surg.* **2023**, *52*, 621–629. [CrossRef] [PubMed]
25. Walia, A.; Lee, J.J.; Jackson, R.S.; Hardi, A.C.; Bollig, C.A.; Graboyes, E.M.; Zenga, J.; Puram, S.V.; Pipkorn, P. Management of Flap Failure After Head and Neck Reconstruction: A Systematic Review and Meta-analysis. *Otolaryngol. Head Neck Surg.* **2022**, *167*, 224–235. [CrossRef] [PubMed]

Disclaimer/Publisher's Note: The statements, opinions and data contained in all publications are solely those of the individual author(s) and contributor(s) and not of MDPI and/or the editor(s). MDPI and/or the editor(s) disclaim responsibility for any injury to people or property resulting from any ideas, methods, instructions or products referred to in the content.

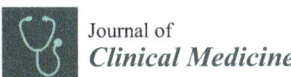 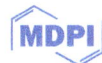

Review

Expanding the Armamentarium of Donor Sites in Microvascular Head and Neck Reconstruction

Z-Hye Lee, Ana Canzi, Jessie Yu and Edward I. Chang *

Department of Plastic Surgery, University of Texas MD Anderson Cancer Center, 1400 Pressler Street, Houston, TX 77030, USA
* Correspondence: eichang@mdanderson.org; Tel.: +1-713-794-1247

Abstract: The field of microsurgical head and neck reconstruction has witnessed tremendous advancements in recent years. While the historic goals of reconstruction were simply to maximize flap survival, optimizing both aesthetic and functional outcomes has now become the priority. With an increased understanding of perforator anatomy, improved technology in instruments and microscopes, and high flap success rates, the reconstructive microsurgeon can push the envelope in harvesting and designing the ideal flap to aid patients following tumor extirpation. Furthermore, with improvements in cancer treatment leading to improved patient survival and prognosis, it becomes increasingly important to have a broader repertoire of donor sites. The present review aims to provide a review of newly emerging soft tissue flap options in head and neck reconstruction. While certainly a number of bony flap options also exist, the present review will focus on soft tissue flaps that can be harvested reliably from a variety of alternate donor sites. From the upper extremity, the ulnar forearm as well as the lateral arm, and from the lower extremity, the profunda artery perforator, medial sural artery perforator, and superficial circumflex iliac perforator flaps will be discussed, and we will provide details to aid reconstructive microsurgeons in incorporating these alternative flaps into their armamentarium.

Keywords: head and neck reconstruction; microvascular reconstruction; workhorse-free flaps

Citation: Lee, Z.-H.; Canzi, A.; Yu, J.; Chang, E.I. Expanding the Armamentarium of Donor Sites in Microvascular Head and Neck Reconstruction. *J. Clin. Med.* **2024**, *13*, 1311. https://doi.org/10.3390/jcm13051311

Academic Editors: Boban M. Erovic and Matteo Alicandri-Ciufelli

Received: 26 December 2023
Revised: 3 February 2024
Accepted: 23 February 2024
Published: 26 February 2024

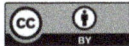

Copyright: © 2024 by the authors. Licensee MDPI, Basel, Switzerland. This article is an open access article distributed under the terms and conditions of the Creative Commons Attribution (CC BY) license (https://creativecommons.org/licenses/by/4.0/).

1. Introduction

Microvascular head and neck reconstruction has advanced tremendously over the years with high flap success rates often over 95% at most high-volume centers [1–3]. With the high success rates that can be achieved in the current era, the reconstructive demands have also increased. The goals of reconstruction have progressed well beyond simply preventing thrombosis and total flap loss. The microsurgeon is now more than ever tasked with optimizing the aesthetic and functional outcomes for patients undergoing tumor extirpation. While the overwhelming majority of defects can be reliably reconstructed using the standard workhorse flaps such as the radial forearm, the anterolateral thigh (ALT), and the latissimus dorsi flap, circumstances can arise where alternate donor sites may be necessary. With the improvements in cancer treatment and patient survival, patients may develop recurrent disease, develop complications following radiation, or may undergo such extensive resections that multiple flaps are needed [4]. As such, the reconstructive microsurgeon should become familiar with alternate donor sites in the setting that the standard workhorse donor sites are unavailable [5].

While the radial forearm remains one of the most reliable flaps with a long pedicle and provides thin pliable tissue, the need for a skin graft to the donor site or radial dominant perfusion to the hand may necessitate an alternative donor site. In the Western population where an increasing body mass index and obesity are increasingly common, the ALT may be prohibitively thick, while in other circumstances, when patients are malnourished and suffer significant weight loss, perhaps donor sites with more volume are warranted. The present article aims to provide a review and synopsis of some donor sites that have been gaining popularity and may benefit surgeons performing high-volume microvascular head and neck reconstruction. The review aims to provide a synopsis of the ulnar forearm, lateral arm, profunda artery perforator (PAP), medial sural artery perforator (MSAP), and superficial circumflex iliac perforator (SCIP) flaps, focusing on anatomy and pearls and pitfalls to the utilization of these flaps in head and neck reconstruction.

2. Ulnar Forearm Flap

While the radial forearm continues to remain one of the most popular donor sites, in circumstances when the patient is radial dominant or perhaps arterial catheters have been placed into the radial artery, a flap based on the ulnar artery is a reliable option to consider. However, in other circumstances, one may opt to use the ulnar donor site as the primary option to design a flap with slightly more volume or harvest a flap that is less hair-bearing. In these circumstances, an Allen test should also be performed to ensure that perfusion to the hand will not be compromised with the sacrifice of the ulnar artery [6].

The ulnar forearm flap can be harvested distally just proximal to the wrist crease, similar to the design of a radial forearm flap. The artery is readily palpable or can be identified with a handheld Doppler to orient the flap so that it is centered over the ulnar artery. The flap is raised as a fasciocutaneous flap, again similar to the harvest of the radial forearm flap. A distally based ulnar fasciocutaneous flap will provide a longer pedicle; however, designing the flap more distally in this fashion will lead to exposure of the flexor digitorum superficialis (FDS) and the flexor carpi ulnaris (FCU) tendons that can become exposed in the setting that the skin graft has poor take [7]. The flap harvest should therefore aim to preserve the fascia over the tendons to minimize wound healing complications of the skin graft over the tendons.

Alternatively, the flap can be harvested as a perforator flap which has also been proven to be extremely reliable. The ulnar artery perforator (UAP) flap is harvested more proximally than its fasciocutaneous counterpart since the perforators arise more proximally [8,9]. The distal extent of the flap is typically oriented approximately five centimeters proximal to the pisiform along an axis from the pisiform to the medial epicondyle (Figure 1). By harvesting the flap more proximally, the average pedicle length is approximately 7.1 cm; however, this reduces the risks of tendon exposure and compromised take of the skin graft. Perforators have been reliably mapped using the pisiform as a landmark where the A, B, and C perforators arise 7 cm, 11 cm, and 15 cm from the pisiform, respectively. The flap dissection starts on the radial side and is harvested in a suprafascial plane until the dissection proceeds to the FDS and FCU tendons from the radial and ulnar sides, respectively. At this time, the dissection must proceed in a subfascial plane to include the pedicle and perforators in the flap. During the dissection, careful attention must be paid to avoid injury to the ulnar nerve which is intimately adjacent to the ulnar vessels (Figure 2).

Studies examining outcomes using an ulnar forearm flap have proven to have equally high success rates and equivalent post-operative speech and swallowing function when compared to the radial forearm flap [10]. Not surprisingly, studies examining donor site morbidity have also demonstrated similar risks of complications compared to the radial forearm donor site [11–13]. Some studies have even found superior outcomes with the ulnar forearm donor site compared to its radial counterpart [14].

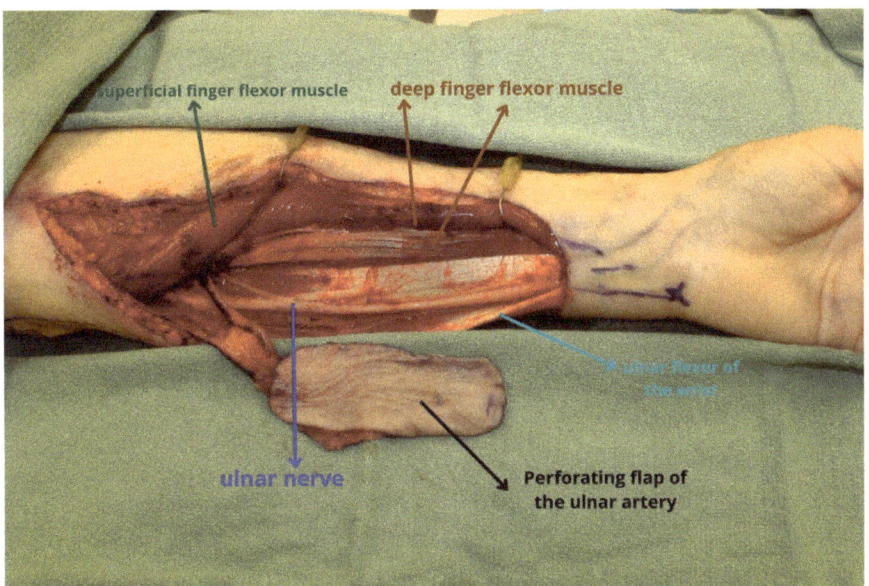

Figure 1. The ulnar artery perforator flap is based on perforators arising from the ulnar artery and is harvested more proximally to avoid issues with tendon exposure in the setting of poor skin graft take. As noted, the flap is on the ulnar aspect of the forearm which is often less hair-baring, but the pedicle length is shorter than the radial forearm flap.

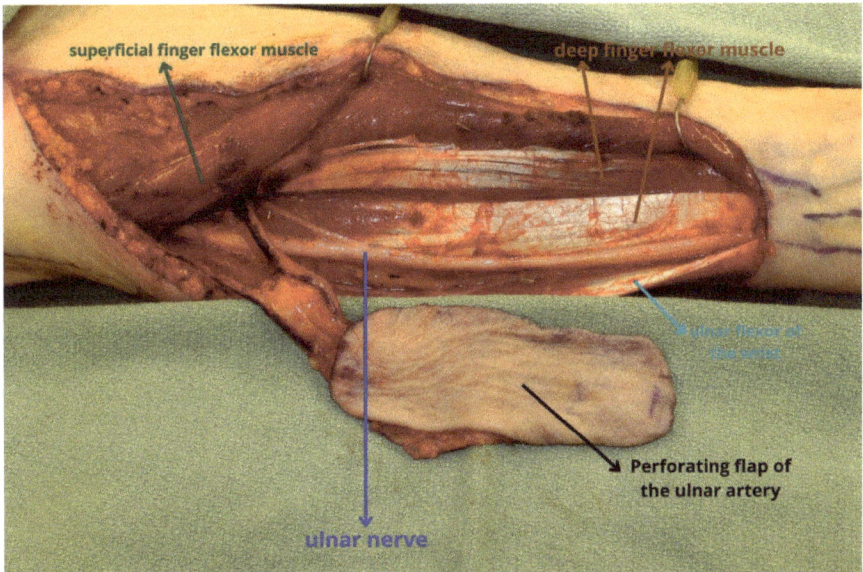

Figure 2. During dissection, it is critical to avoid injury to the ulnar nerve which runs in close proximity to the pedicle as depicted. The soft tissue flap is ideally suited for the reconstruction of partial glossectomy, buccal mucosal, or palatal defects. The present flap was utilized for reconstruction of a partial glossectomy defect. Dissection of the pedicle can be performed more proximally to gain additional pedicle length, but flap selection should consider the availability of recipient vessels.

3. Lateral Arm and Lateral Forearm Flap

The lateral arm represents a unique donor site option that permits the harvest of a flap of variable thickness that can be tailored based on the extent of the defect [15]. For many head and neck defects, the lateral arm also provides a comparable color match to facial skin compared to the thighs (Figure 3). Similar to the ulnar forearm donor site, a lateral arm flap can be harvested as a fasciocutaneous flap or a perforator flap. Also like the ulnar forearm flap, a true lateral arm perforator flap has a shorter pedicle compared to a more distally oriented fasciocutaneous flap. While the flap can be harvested more proximally as a perforator flap or more distally as a fasciocutaneous flap, the microsurgeon should be cognizant of the relatively smaller caliber artery which is typically less than 2 mm as well as the proximity of the radial nerve to the pedicle (Figure 4).

The lateral arm perforator (LAP) flap is harvested from the upper lateral arm and is a true perforator flap. The perforator anatomy is remarkably reliable, similar to other perforator flaps that have been described [16]. Using the landmarks of the deltoid insertion and the lateral epicondyle, the perforator locations can typically be found 7 cm, 10 cm, and 12 cm from the deltoid insertion. The flap dissection should begin from the posterior side. The dissection should be subfascial progressing from posterior to anterior towards the septum between the triceps and biceps muscles. The flap is often of an intermediate thickness between the ALT and a forearm-based flap [17]. Another advantage of the LAP flap is the opportunity to create a sensate flap as the lateral antebrachial cutaneous nerve often needs to be divided during perforator and pedicle dissection. As a trade-off, there can be an area of numbness in the donor site along the dermatomal distribution of the nerve. The LAP pedicle is considerably shorter compared to a more distally based fasciocutaneous flap which will be discussed later. On average, the length of the pedicle is approximately 7 cm, and the reconstructive microsurgeon should be conscious of the pedicle length during flap selection [16].

A more distally based lateral arm flap has been named the extended lateral arm flap or the lateral forearm flap which is a more distally based flap that can be taken over the lateral epicondyle [18]. A flap harvested this distally is often very thin and pliable and may be as thin or thinner than a traditional forearm-based flap [19]. The more distally oriented fasciocutaneous flap is centered over the distal extent of the vascular pedicle which significantly increases the pedicle length. The maximum width of the flap that can be harvested is based on the "pinch test" but is typically less than 6 cm to allow for primary closure of the donor site. Consequently, an added benefit of the lateral forearm is that it allows for the harvesting of a thin, pliable flap without the need for a skin graft to the donor site. Similar to the LAP, the cutaneous nerve can also be harvested with the flap to create a sensate flap, or the nerve can also be preserved in many circumstances to avoid numbness in the lateral arm dermatome.

The closure of the donor site for the lateral arm flaps should be carried out without tension and without re-approximation of the muscle or closure of the deep layers. A tight closure can result in radial nerve palsy with post-operative swelling that has catastrophic consequences if the radial nerve deficits do not resolve [20]. Thus, even if the flap harvest is performed using a no-touch technique, paying careful attention to protect the nerve, a tight closure can still result in neurologic deficits. While suboptimal, a skin graft to the donor site is preferable to a radial nerve deficit.

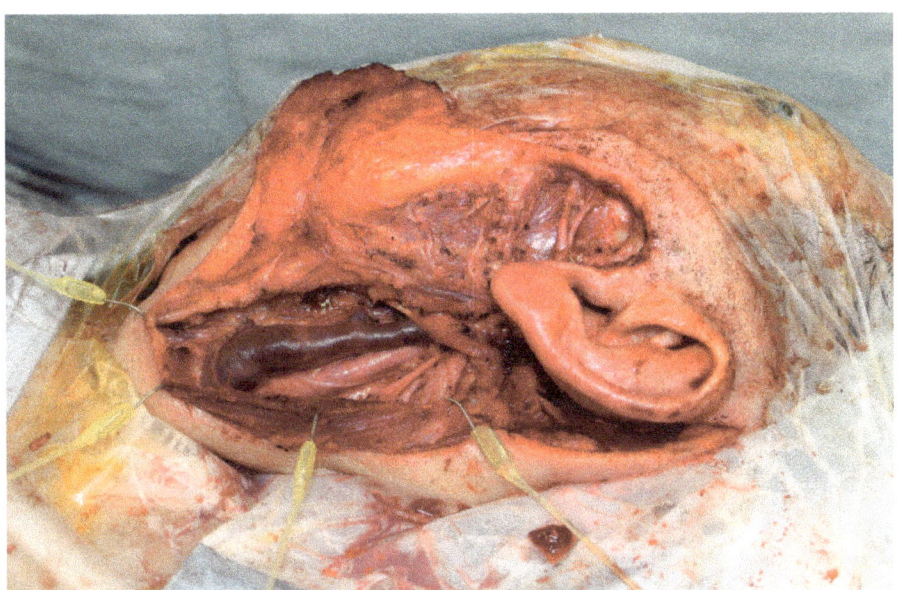

Figure 3. Parotidectomy defect with preservation of the facial nerve but with a significant skin resection. The lateral arm donor site often provides a suitable color match to the facial skin and can be harvested more proximally or distally based on the thickness needed.

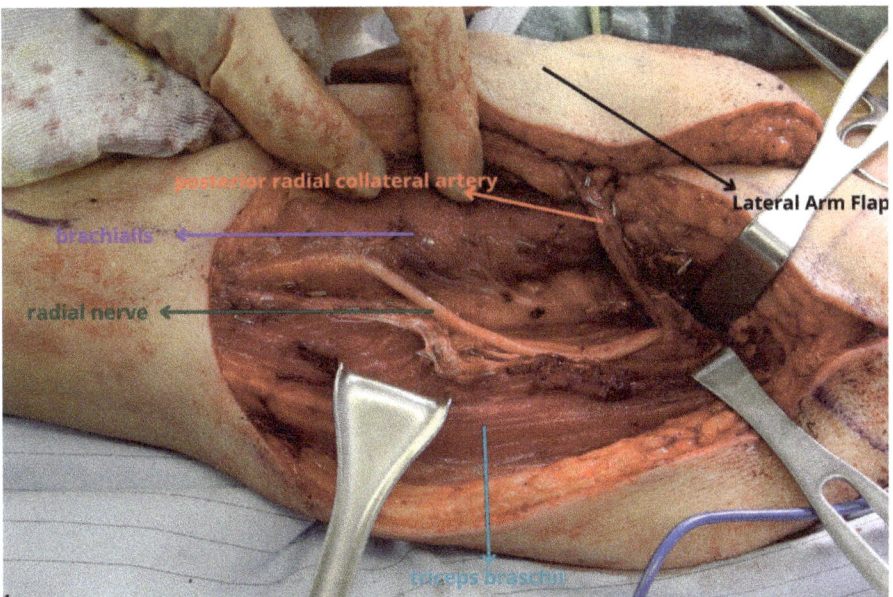

Figure 4. The radial nerve lies in close proximity to the pedicle and must be carefully protected during dissection. The patient's thigh was too thick to use for the parotidectomy defect which is more common in the Western population. The lateral arm flap is well-suited as a flap that is often intermediate in thickness. Designing the flap more proximally as shown will provide more thickness while a more distally oriented flap will provide thinner tissue but allow for a longer pedicle. The design of the flap can be adjusted based on the extent of the defect and the need for more volume.

4. Profunda Artery Perforator Flap

The profunda artery perforator (PAP) flap has been popularized in the United States as the secondary workhorse flap for autologous breast reconstruction [21,22], but the donor site also represents a reliable option for the reconstruction of head and neck defects [23]. While most PAP flaps performed for breast reconstruction are typically harvested in a transverse orientation, the perforator anatomy is much more reliable in a vertically oriented flap. The perforator anatomy again has proven to be remarkably reliable and likely more reliable than the ALT, which can have tremendous variation and in some circumstances may not have any suitable perforators at all. For many head and neck patients who suffer from weight loss due to the extensive tumor burden, pain, trismus, or the sequelae of previous radiation, the PAP can provide tissue that is thicker than the ALT (Figures 5 and 6) [24–26]. The length of the flap can be tailored to the size of the defect, but the width that can be harvested is variable from patient to patient and is dependent on the laxity in the donor site. In some instances, flaps as wide or wider than 10 cm can be harvested while still allowing for primary closure of the donor site.

Based on the groin crease, perforators again can be reliably found at 8 cm, 13 cm, and 18 cm from the crease [27]. While the proximal-most perforator is often present, it is often not the largest perforator which tends to be more distal. Therefore, if one plans to harvest the flap in a transverse orientation, imaging studies are recommended for the novice microsurgeon to confirm the presence of a suitable perforator to allow the harvest of a transverse PAP flap. The dissection begins from the anterior edge of the flap and should proceed posterior to the gracilis muscle where the fascia overlying the adductor magnus is incised to identify the perforators. Since the perforators tend to arise from the profunda femoris vessels in a segmental fashion, the microsurgeon should be aware that it is difficult to design a PAP with two separate skin islands. Harvesting a chimeric PAP is possible by taking a portion of the adductor magnus if a large muscle branch is identified arising from the same perforator. In contrast to other chimeric flaps, the fasciocutaneous skin component and the muscle are typically very close to each other, which limits and restricts the mobility of each component.

The pedicle length tends to be somewhat deceptive as the dissection is performed through an intramuscular course to its takeoff from the source vessels. The trajectory can result in a pedicle that nears 12–15 cm in situ; however, upon ligation of the vessels, the pedicle length tends to retract considerably and often only provides a pedicle length of up to 8–10 cm. The artery is generally smaller compared to the ALT, typically approximately 2 mm, while the vein is usually a reasonable caliber similar to the ALT.

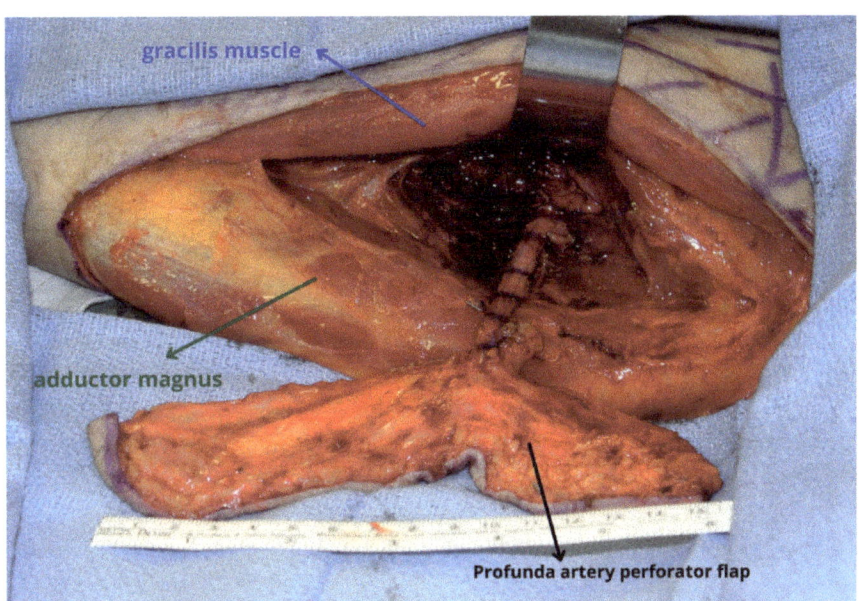

Figure 5. Profunda artery perforator flap harvested based on perforators arising from the profunda femoris artery with suitable pedicle length when the pedicle is dissected to its origin from the profunda femoris artery. To gain a longer pedicle and a larger caliber artery, the dissection should be performed to the takeoff from the profunda femoris artery. Retraction of the gracilis muscle is necessary to perform the more proximal dissection to the origin of the pedicle.

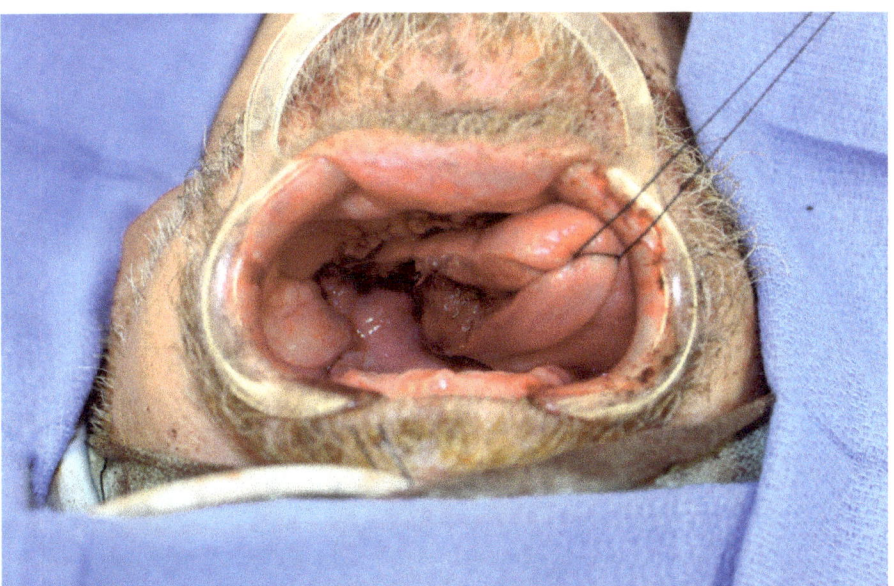

Figure 6. A defect that was reconstructed using the MSAP flap. Hemiglossectomy defect that could be reconstructed with any number of potential donor sites. However, using an upper extremity flap often requires sequential harvest after the resection is completed. Using a thinner donor site from the lower extremity allows for simultaneous harvest and can shorten the operating time.

5. Medial Sural Artery Perforator Flap

The medial sural artery perforator (MSAP) flap is another alternate donor site that is gaining popularity [28,29]. While it is more commonly used for limb salvage and extremity reconstruction, the flap also represents a potential donor site when thinner tissue is needed for head and neck reconstruction (Figures 6 and 7). While the tissue may be somewhat thicker than an upper extremity flap, the tissue is still typically thinner and more pliable than the thigh [30–32]. One potential advantage of the MSAP over the upper extremity flaps is the opportunity for simultaneous harvest in conjunction with the resection [32]. Thus, a two-team approach can reduce the operative time whereas harvest of a forearm flap or the lateral arm is generally difficult to perform at the same as with the resecting team. Unfortunately, flap harvest is limited to a width of approximately 6 cm but can vary based on the patient's body habitus to allow for primary closure of the donor site. While a skin graft may be suboptimal, a tight closure should be avoided to avoid the risks of compartment syndrome.

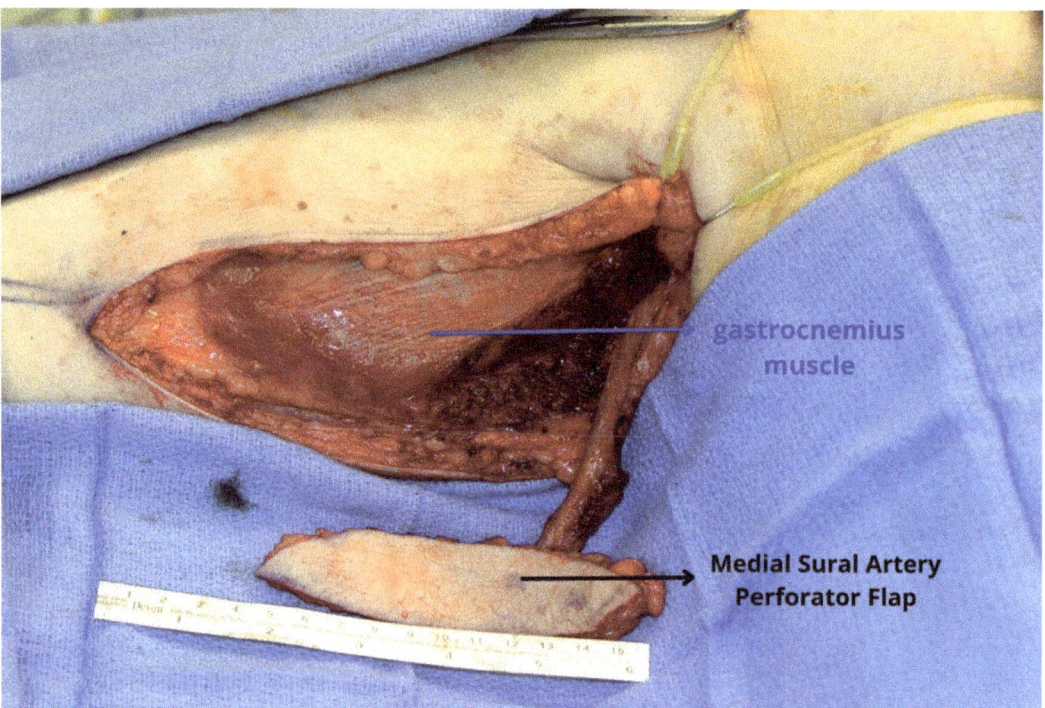

Figure 7. The medial sural artery perforator flap harvested from the calf region provides a suitably thin, pliable tissue to reconstruct the hemiglossectomy defect. The pedicle length is quite variable with the MSAP flap, and while a 10–12 cm pedicle is possible, this is rather inconsistent from one patient to another.

The greatest limitation of the MSAP is the freestyle nature of the flap harvest [33]. While recommendations use the landmarks of the midline of the popliteal crease and the medial malleolus 8–18 cm along this axis is marginal [34,35], most microsurgeons still advocate using a hand-held Doppler to locate perforators before making the skin incision; however, an ultrasound can greatly simplify the flap design and harvest. Most times, the perforators are located posterior to the axis, but due to the freestyle nature of this flap, there is a possibility that the perforators may be located anteriorly. Some have performed endoscopic-assisted MSAP harvests to visualize the perforator using a minimally invasive incision to aid in flap design [36].

The location of the perforator will dictate the pedicle length, which, again, can be quite variable, but for a distally located perforator, pedicle lengths of 10–12 cm can be harvested. Another reflection of the freestyle nature of the flap is the vessel caliber, which, again, is quite variable. If the perforator arises from the main medial sural artery, the vessels are sizable, but often the perforator may arise from a secondary branch of the main medial sural vessels, leading to vessels that are on average less than 2 mm in diameter. In a virgin neck, an ample number of potential recipients are available, and selection of the superior thyroid artery or another smaller caliber artery may represent a more suitable recipient than one that creates an unfavorable size mismatch [37].

6. Superficial Circumflex Iliac Perforator Flap

Finally, the superficial circumflex iliac perforator (SCIP) flap is another donor site that is gaining popularity for head and neck reconstruction [38]. The SCIP or groin flap has long been a workhorse flap for reconstructive surgeons and has been popularized for extremity reconstructive and limb salvage [38–40]. With the increased comfort and understanding of the anatomy, indications for the SCIP are rapidly expanding. Its use is well-documented in extremity reconstruction, particularly diabetic foot wounds as well as in the growing field of lymphedema surgery; however, its utility in head and neck reconstruction remains to be elucidated. The majority of cases have used the SCIP for the reconstruction of relatively smaller intraoral defects such as for partial glossectomy or buccal mucosal defects [41–44].

In the hands of experienced microsurgeons, the SCIP flap provides reliable thin tissue that can also be tailored as a super-thin flap or a thicker flap if both the deep and superficial branches of the superficial circumflex iliac vessels are incorporated. With the increased comfort in flap design and dissection, some authors have expanded the utility of the flap by including a portion of the iliac crest, thereby creating another option for an osteocutaneous flap (Figure 8) [45,46]. The flap can be harvested in conjunction with the resection, thereby shortening the operative time, and has minimal donor site morbidity as the donor site can be closed primarily without the need for a skin graft, leaving a well-concealed scar in the inguinal region. However, while the use of the SCIP is gradually expanding, the anatomy and dissection can pose some challenges to the novice microsurgeon. For many, the incorporation of preoperative or intraoperative ultrasound to define the vascular anatomy has greatly simplified flap harvest [47,48]. Other limitations of the SCIP flap include factors such as the pedicle length, which is relatively shorter with an average length of approximately 5 cm, and the caliber of the vessels, particularly the artery, which tend to be considerably smaller compared to some other donor sites, occasionally only one millimeter in size.

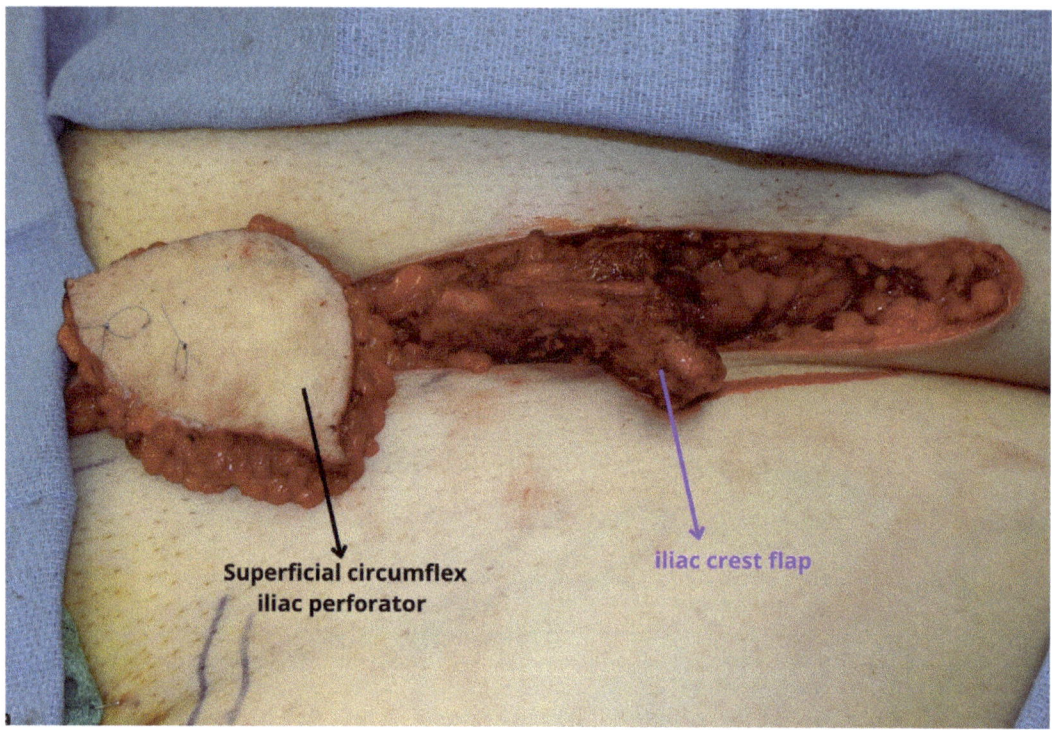

Figure 8. The skin paddle overlying an iliac crest flap is challenging to include with the bone, but in the setting that a skin paddle cannot be harvested with the bone based on the deep circumflex iliac artery (DCIA), a fasciocutaneous flap can be harvested based on the superficial circumflex iliac artery demonstrated here. The thickness of the superficial circumflex iliac perforator (SCIP) flap is variable based on the patient's body habitus and may be thicker in the Western population. While difficult to appreciate in the figure, the pedicle length and caliber of the vessels are much smaller compared to other flaps and should be considered by the reconstructive surgeon prior to using this flap.

7. Discussion

The field of reconstructive microsurgery has revolutionized the treatment of cancer where patients previously destined for palliation, amputation, or lifelong disfigurement can now be reconstructed with high success rates and minimal complications. With the advances in technology and increased experience with microsurgery, the reconstructive microsurgeon now must consider the functional and aesthetic outcomes rather than simply focusing on flap survival. Furthermore, with the tremendous gains in cancer care, patients previously not considered surgical candidates are now able to undergo tumor extirpation with curative intent, and the onus falls on the reconstructive surgeon to optimize their quality of life. Along the same vein, modern oncologic treatments have also improved prognosis and increased patient survival, so the microsurgeon can be expected to encounter more patients who either develop recurrence or need to undergo salvage operation with another free tissue transfer. Similarly, with improved survival, patients may also suffer late complications such as hardware exposure and again need another microvascular reconstruction [49–51]. Under these circumstances, the reconstructive surgeon must have a broader armamentarium of flap options to be able to reconstruct these secondary defects and provide the most optimal functional and aesthetic outcomes for patients.

While there is little debate that the radial forearm, ALT, and latissimus dorsi flaps are the traditional workhorse flaps, there are also limitations to consider. The need for skin grafting and donor site morbidity of the radial forearm and the unpredictable perforator anatomy of the ALT are common complaints at both donor sites, while the latissimus dorsi typically requires harvest in a lateral decubitus position. In contrast, the alternative options presented can all be closed primarily, obviating the need for a skin graft except for the ulnar forearm donor site, although, in certain circumstances, even the ulnar forearm can be closed primarily. The PAP perforator anatomy has proven to be more reliable and consistent compared to the ALT. However, while there are certainly advantages and benefits to these alternative flaps, there are also significant limitations that must be considered.

For the majority of the alternate donor sites, the pedicle length is usually shorter, and the caliber of the artery is typically smaller when compared to the radial forearm, ALT, or latissimus dorsi flaps [5]. The vein however is typically an adequate size comparable to the diameter of the main workhorse flaps. Unfortunately, the size of the vessels cannot be modified, but the length can potentially be adjusted by harvesting and designing a more distal flap as in the ulnar forearm or the lateral arm to obtain a longer pedicle. In the setting of a redo sequential free flap or in the setting of salvage after total flap loss, a longer pedicle to reach more distant recipient vessels may be necessary to avoid the need for a vein graft. In certain circumstances, a vein graft cannot be avoided, but efforts should be made to avoid them if possible, given the higher risks of complications [52,53].

Perhaps the greatest area of consideration is whether these alternate flaps should replace the current workhorse flaps. With the increased experience and comfort with perforator flaps and smaller caliber vessels, the success rates of alternate flap donor sites and workhorse flaps are equivalent. Given the equivalent success rates, consideration perhaps should be given to using the alternate flaps as a first-line option, thereby preserving the traditional workhorse flaps in the setting of recurrent disease, flap loss, or post-operative complications. In the virgin neck when a plethora of recipient vessels are available, the shorter pedicle length that is often the Achilles' heel of the alternate flaps becomes less of an issue. Perhaps in the current era of microvascular head and neck reconstruction, a paradigm shift may be warranted to consider using the lateral arm, PAP, MSAP, or SCIP flaps as the primary means of reconstruction. At the authors' institution, this is becoming an increasingly popular approach where the lateral forearm flap has largely supplanted the radial or ulnar forearm flaps to avoid donor site morbidity and the need for skin grafting.

Ultimately, the reconstructive surgeon must consider all factors when discussing the available donor site options with patients. The reconstructive surgeon must assess the available donor sites, which can vary tremendously in different patient populations as Western populations tend to be more obese, precluding them from certain donor sites that are more common in Asia. Aside from the donor site itself, the surgeon must also consider the defect and select the most appropriate flap to achieve the best possible outcome. For instance, for an extensive through-and-through defect, if a flap with multiple components is needed, the ALT still represents the most reliable option. The ALT can be harvested, potentially with multiple skin paddles, and can easily also include muscle if necessary [54]. While a chimeric flap can also be designed for the PAP or the MSAP, this is often more challenging and limited due to the restrictions in mobility and length that can be obtained for each chimeric component. Finally, the surgeon must have the insight and experience to determine which donor site can be used safely and reliably. For a surgeon who has never performed one of the alternative flaps and has a complex defect in a previously operated and radiated neck, perhaps using a traditional workhorse flap would be the most prudent.

8. Conclusions

Microvascular head and neck reconstruction is an exceedingly challenging subspecialty in microsurgery that forces the surgeon to incorporate all of the principles of reconstructive surgery to optimize the patient's aesthetics and function. While most defects can be successfully reconstructed with a limited number of free flap donor sites, alternative flaps can expand the armamentarium of reconstructive options in the setting of salvage surgery, flap loss, or when the traditional workhorse flaps are not available.

Author Contributions: Conceptualization, Z.-H.L., A.C., J.Y. and E.I.C.; validation, Z.-H.L., A.C., J.Y. and E.I.C.; writing—original draft preparation, A.C. and E.I.C.; writing—review and editing, Z.-H.L., A.C., J.Y. and E.I.C.; supervision, E.I.C. All authors have read and agreed to the published version of the manuscript.

Funding: No funding was received for the production of this work.

Institutional Review Board Statement: Ethical review and approval were waived for this study as this was a Review Article and did not include patient specific data.

Informed Consent Statement: Patient consent was waived as no identifying features were included in any images that would violate patient confidentiality.

Data Availability Statement: No new data were created in the production of this work.

Conflicts of Interest: No financial affiliations or conflicts of interest involved in the production of this work.

References

1. Wong, C.H.; Wei, F.C. Microsurgical free flap in head and neck reconstruction. *Head Neck* **2010**, *32*, 1236–1245. [CrossRef]
2. Mücke, T.; Ritschl, L.M.; Roth, M.; Güll, F.D.; Rau, A.; Grill, S.; Kesting, M.R.; Wolff, K.D.; Loeffelbein, D.J. Predictors of free flap loss in the head and neck region: A four-year retrospective study with 451 microvascular transplants at a single centre. *J. Craniomaxillofac. Surg.* **2016**, *44*, 1292–1298. [CrossRef]
3. Pellini, R.; De Virgilio, A.; Mercante, G.; Pichi, B.; Manciocco, V.; Marchesi, P.; Ferreli, F.; Spriano, G. Vastus lateralis myofascial free flap in tongue reconstruction. *Acta Otorhinolaryngol. Ital.* **2016**, *36*, 321–325. [CrossRef]
4. Chang, E.I.; Hanasono, M.M.; Butler, C.E. Management of Unfavorable Outcomes in Head and Neck Free Flap Reconstruction: Experience-Based Lessons from the MD Anderson Cancer Center. *Clin. Plast. Surg.* **2016**, *43*, 653–667. [CrossRef]
5. Chang, E.I. Alternate Soft-Tissue Free Flaps for Head and Neck Reconstruction: The Next Generation of Workhorse Flaps. *Plast. Reconstr. Surg.* **2023**, *152*, 184–193. [CrossRef]
6. Wood, J.W.; Broussard, K.C.; Burkey, B. Preoperative testing for radial forearm free flaps to reduce donor site morbidity. *JAMA Otolaryngol. Head Neck Surg.* **2013**, *139*, 183–186. [CrossRef]
7. Kantar, R.S.; Rifkin, W.J.; Cammarata, M.J.; Jacoby, A.; Farber, S.J.; Diaz-Siso, J.R.; Ceradini, D.J.; Rodriguez, E.D. Appraisal of the Free Ulnar Flap Versatility in Craniofacial Soft-tissue Reconstruction. *Plast. Reconstr. Surg. Glob. Open.* **2018**, *6*, e1863. [CrossRef] [PubMed]
8. Yu, P.; Chang, E.I.; Selber, J.C.; Hanasono, M.M. Perforator patterns of the ulnar artery perforator flap. *Plast. Reconstr. Surg.* **2012**, *129*, 213–220. [CrossRef] [PubMed]
9. Ishiko, M.; Yano, K.; Onode, E.; Takamatsu, K. Identification of Ulnar Artery Perforators Using Color Doppler Ultrasonography. *J. Reconstr. Microsurg.* **2020**, *36*, 667–672. [CrossRef] [PubMed]
10. Antony, A.K.; Hootnick, J.L.; Antony, A.K. Ulnar forearm free flaps in head and neck reconstruction: Systematic review of the literature and a case report. *Microsurgery* **2014**, *34*, 68–75. [CrossRef]
11. Hekner, D.D.; Abbink, J.H.; van Es, R.J.; Rosenberg, A.; Koole, R.; Van Cann, E.M. Donor-site morbidity of the radial forearm free flap versus the ulnar forearm free flap. *Plast. Reconstr. Surg.* **2013**, *132*, 387–393. [CrossRef]
12. Chang, E.I.; Liu, J. Prospective Comparison of Donor-Site Morbidity following Radial Forearm and Ulnar Artery Perforator Flap Harvest. *Plast. Reconstr. Surg.* **2020**, *145*, 1267–1274. [CrossRef]
13. Thiem, D.G.E.; Siegberg, F.; Römer, P.; Blatt, S.; Pabst, A.; Heimes, D.; Al-Nawas, B.; Kämmerer, P.W. Long-Term Donor Site Morbidity and Flap Perfusion Following Radial versus Ulnar Forearm Free Flap-A Randomized Controlled Prospective Clinical Trial. *J. Clin. Med.* **2022**, *11*, 3601. [CrossRef] [PubMed]
14. Xu, Q.; Chen, P.L.; Liu, Y.H.; Wang, S.M.; Xu, Z.F.; Feng, C.J. Comparing donor site morbidity between radial and ulnar forearm free flaps: A meta-analysis. *Br. J. Oral. Maxillofac. Surg.* **2022**, *60*, 547–553. [CrossRef] [PubMed]
15. Marques Faria, J.C.; Rodrigues, M.L.; Scopel, G.P.; Kowalski, L.P.; Ferreira, M.C. The versatility of the free lateral arm flap in head and neck soft tissue reconstruction: Clinical experience of 210 cases. *J. Plast. Reconstr. Aesthet. Surg.* **2008**, *61*, 172–179. [CrossRef] [PubMed]
16. Chang, E.I.; Ibrahim, A.; Papazian, N.; Jurgus, A.; Nguyen, A.T.; Suami, H.; Yu, P. Perforator Mapping and Optimizing Design of the Lateral Arm Flap: Anatomy Revisited and Clinical Experience. *Plast. Reconstr. Surg.* **2016**, *138*, 300e–306e. [CrossRef] [PubMed]
17. Busnardo, F.F.; Coltro, P.S.; Olivan, M.V.; Faes, J.C.; Lavor, E.; Ferreira, M.C.; Rodrigues, A.J., Jr.; Gemperli, R. Anatomical comparison among the anterolateral thigh, the parascapular, and the lateral arm flaps. *Microsurgery* **2015**, *35*, 387–392. [CrossRef] [PubMed]
18. Shuck, J.; Chang, E.I.; Mericli, A.F.; Gross, N.D.; Hanasono, M.M.; Garvey, P.B.; Yu, P.; Largo, R.D. Free Lateral Forearm Flap in Head and Neck Reconstruction: An Attractive Alternative to the Radial Forearm Flap. *Plast. Reconstr. Surg.* **2020**, *146*, 446e–450e. [CrossRef]

19. Danker, S.; Shuck, J.W.; Taher, A.; Mujtaba, B.; Chang, E.I.; Chu, C.K.; Liu, J.; Garvey, P.B.; Hanna, E.; Yu, P.; et al. The lateral forearm flap versus traditional upper extremity flaps: A comparison of donor site morbidity and flap thickness. *Head Neck* **2023**, *45*, 2413–2423. [CrossRef]
20. Contrera, K.J.; Hassan, A.M.; Shuck, J.W.; Bobian, M.; Ha, A.Y.; Chang, E.I.; Garvey, P.B.; Roubaud, M.S.; Lee, Z.H.; Hanasono, M.M.; et al. Outcomes for 160 Consecutive Lateral Arm Free Flaps for Head and Neck Reconstruction. *Otolaryngol. Head Neck Surg.* **2023**. [CrossRef]
21. Chu, C.K.; Largo, R.D.; Lee, Z.H.; Adelman, D.M.; Egro, F.; Winocour, S.; Reece, E.M.; Selber, J.C.; Butler, C.E. Introduction of the L-PAP Flap: Bipedicled, Conjoined, and Stacked Thigh-Based Flaps for Autologous Breast Reconstruction. *Plast. Reconstr. Surg.* **2023**, *152*, 1005e–1010e. [CrossRef]
22. Cohen, Z.; Azoury, S.C.; Matros, E.; Nelson, J.A.; Allen, R.J., Jr. Modern Approaches to Alternative Flap-Based Breast Reconstruction: Profunda Artery Perforator Flap. *Clin. Plast. Surg.* **2023**, *50*, 289–299. [CrossRef] [PubMed]
23. Largo, R.D.; Bhadkamkar, M.A.; Asaad, M.; Chu, C.K.; Garvey, P.B.; Butler, C.E.; Yu, P.; Hanasono, M.M.; Chang, E.I. The Profunda Artery Perforator Flap: A Versatile Option for Head and Neck Reconstruction. *Plast. Reconstr. Surg.* **2021**, *147*, 1401–1412. [CrossRef] [PubMed]
24. Ismail, T.; Padilla, P.; Kurlander, D.E.; Corkum, J.P.; Hanasono, M.M.; Garvey, P.B.; Chang, E.I.; Yu, P.; Largo, R.D. Profunda Artery Perforator Flap Tongue Reconstruction: An Effective and Safe Alternative to the Anterolateral Thigh Flap. *Plast. Reconstr. Surg.* **2023**. [CrossRef] [PubMed]
25. Liu, S.W.; Hanick, A.L.; Meleca, J.B.; Roskies, M.; Hadford, S.P.; Genther, D.J.; Ciolek, P.J.; Lamarre, E.D.; Ku, J.A. The profunda artery perforator flap for head and neck reconstruction. *Am. J. Otolaryngol.* **2023**, *44*, 103772. [CrossRef] [PubMed]
26. Yao, C.M.K.; Jozaghi, Y.; Danker, S.; Karami, R.; Asaad, M.; Lai, S.Y.; Hanna, E.Y.; Esmaeli, B.; Gidley, P.W.; Chang, E.I. The combined profunda artery perforator-gracilis flap for immediate facial reanimation and resurfacing of the radical parotidectomy defect. *Microsurgery* **2023**, *43*, 309–315. [CrossRef] [PubMed]
27. Largo, R.D.; Chu, C.K.; Chang, E.I.; Liu, J.; Abu-Ghname, A.; Wang, H.; Schaverien, M.V.; Mericli, A.F.; Hanasono, M.M.; Yu, P. Perforator Mapping of the Profunda Artery Perforator Flap: Anatomy and Clinical Experience. *Plast. Reconstr. Surg.* **2020**, *146*, 1135–1145. [CrossRef]
28. Deek, N.F.A.; Hsiao, J.C.; Do, N.T.; Kao, H.K.; Hsu, C.C.; Lin, C.H.; Lin, C.H. The Medial Sural Artery Perforator Flap: Lessons Learned from 200 Consecutive Cases. *Plast. Reconstr. Surg.* **2020**, *146*, 630e–641e. [CrossRef] [PubMed]
29. Daar, D.A.; Abdou, S.A.; Cohen, J.M.; Wilson, S.C.; Levine, J.P. Is the Medial Sural Artery Perforator Flap a New Workhorse Flap? A Systematic Review and Meta-Analysis. *Plast. Reconstr. Surg.* **2019**, *143*, 393e–403e. [CrossRef]
30. Danielian, A.; Cheng, M.Y.; Han, P.S.; Blackwell, K.E.; Kerr, R.P.R. Medial Sural Artery Perforator Flap: A Middle Ground Between Anterolateral Thigh and Radial Forearm Flaps. *Otolaryngol. Head Neck Surg.* **2023**, *169*, 852–857. [CrossRef]
31. Al Omran, Y.; Evans, E.; Jordan, C.; Borg, T.M.; AlOmran, S.; Sepehripour, S.; Akhavani, M.A. The Medial Sural Artery Perforator Flap versus Other Free Flaps in Head and Neck Reconstruction: A Systematic Review. *Arch. Plast. Surg.* **2023**, *50*, 264–273. [CrossRef]
32. Ng, M.J.M.; Goh, C.S.L.; Tan, N.C.; Song, D.H.; Ooi, A.S.H. A Head-to-Head Comparison of the Medial Sural Artery Perforator versus Radial Forearm Flap for Tongue Reconstruction. *J. Reconstr. Microsurg.* **2021**, *37*, 445–452. [CrossRef]
33. Molina, A.R.; Citron, I.; Chinaka, F.; Cascarini, L.; Townley, W.A. Calf Perforator Flaps: A Freestyle Solution for Oral Cavity Reconstruction. *Plast. Reconstr. Surg.* **2017**, *139*, 459–465. [CrossRef] [PubMed]
34. Pease, N.L.; Ong, J.; Townley, W.A. Fixed reference points in mapping medial sural artery perforator location. *J. Plast. Reconstr. Aesthet. Surg.* **2015**, *68*, 589–590. [CrossRef] [PubMed]
35. Dusseldorp, J.R.; Pham, Q.J.; Ngo, Q.; Gianoutsos, M.; Moradi, P. Vascular anatomy of the medial sural artery perforator flap: A new classification system of intra-muscular branching patterns. *J. Plast. Reconstr. Aesthet. Surg.* **2014**, *67*, 1267–1275. [CrossRef] [PubMed]
36. Shen, X.Q.; Lv, Y.; Shen, H.; Lu, H.; Wu, S.C.; Lin, X.J. Endoscope-assisted medial sural artery perforator flap for head and neck reconstruction. *J. Plast. Reconstr. Aesthet. Surg.* **2016**, *69*, 1059–1065. [CrossRef] [PubMed]
37. Taufique, Z.M.; Daar, D.A.; Cohen, L.E.; Thanik, V.D.; Levine, J.P.; Jacobson, A.S. The medial sural artery perforator flap: A better option in complex head and neck reconstruction? *Laryngoscope* **2019**, *129*, 1330–1336. [CrossRef]
38. Altiparmak, M.; Cha, H.G.; Hong, J.P.; Suh, H.P. Superficial Circumflex Iliac Artery Perforator Flap as a Workhorse Flap: Systematic Review and Meta-analysis. *J. Reconstr. Microsurg.* **2020**, *36*, 600–605. [CrossRef]
39. Hong, J.P. The Superficial Circumflex Iliac Artery Perforator Flap in Lower Extremity Reconstruction. *Clin. Plast. Surg.* **2021**, *48*, 225–233. [CrossRef] [PubMed]
40. Carrasco-Lopez, C.; Higueras Suñe, C.; Vila-Poyatos, J.; Garcia Senosian, O.; Priego, D.; Del Rio, M.; Malagon, P.; Huesa, L.; Reina-de-la-Torre, F.; Carrera-Burgaya, A. SCIP flap in high-risk extremity reconstruction: Anatomical study of additional superficial venous patterns and implications in caucasian patients. *J. Plast. Reconstr. Aesthet. Surg.* **2020**, *73*, 1174–1205. [CrossRef]
41. Iida, T.; Mihara, M.; Yoshimatsu, H.; Narushima, M.; Koshima, I. Versatility of the superficial circumflex iliac artery perforator flap in head and neck reconstruction. *Ann. Plast. Surg.* **2014**, *72*, 332–336. [CrossRef] [PubMed]
42. Green, R.; Rahman, K.M.; Owen, S.; Paleri, V.; Adams, J.; Ahmed, O.A.; Ragbir, M. The superficial circumflex iliac artery perforator flap in intra-oral reconstruction. *J. Plast. Reconstr. Aesthet. Surg.* **2013**, *66*, 1683–1687. [CrossRef] [PubMed]

43. Scaglioni, M.F.; Meroni, M.; Fritsche, E.; Rajan, G. Superficial Circumflex Iliac Artery Perforator Flap in Advanced Head and Neck Reconstruction: From Simple to Its Chimeric Patterns and Clinical Experience with 22 Cases. *Plast. Reconstr. Surg.* **2022**, *149*, 721–730. [CrossRef] [PubMed]
44. Hurrell, M.J.L.; Clark, J.R.; Ch'ng, S.; Hubert Low, T.H.; Nguyen, K.M.; Elliott, M.S.; Palme, C.E.; Wykes, J. Comparison between the radial forearm and superficial circumflex iliac artery perforator free flaps for oral soft tissue reconstruction. *Int. J. Oral. Maxillofac. Surg.* **2023**, *52*, 181–187. [CrossRef] [PubMed]
45. Zubler, C.; Lese, I.; Pastor, T.; Attinger, M.; Constantinescu, M.A.; Olariu, R. The osteocutaneous SCIP flap: A detailed description of the surgical technique and retrospective cohort study of consecutive cases in a tertiary European centre. *J. Plast. Reconstr. Aesthet. Surg.* **2023**, *77*, 21–30. [CrossRef] [PubMed]
46. Iida, T.; Narushima, M.; Yoshimatsu, H.; Yamamoto, T.; Araki, J.; Koshima, I. A free vascularised iliac bone flap based on superficial circumflex iliac perforators for head and neck reconstruction. *J. Plast. Reconstr. Aesthet. Surg.* **2013**, *66*, 1596–1599. [CrossRef]
47. Fernandez-Garrido, M.; Nunez-Villaveiran, T.; Zamora, P.; Masia, J.; Leon, X. The extended SCIP flap: An anatomical and clinical study of a new SCIP flap design. *J. Plast. Reconstr. Aesthet. Surg.* **2022**, *75*, 3217–3225. [CrossRef]
48. Yoshimatsu, H.; Yamamoto, T.; Hayashi, A.; Fuse, Y.; Karakawa, R.; Iida, T.; Narushima, M.; Tanakura, K.; Weninger, W.J.; Tzou, C.H.J. Use of the transverse branch of the superficial circumflex iliac artery as a landmark facilitating identification and dissection of the deep branch of the superficial circumflex iliac artery for free flap pedicle: Anatomical study and clinical applications. *Microsurgery* **2019**, *39*, 721–729. [CrossRef]
49. Moratin, J.; Horn, D.; Heinemann, M.; Metzger, K.; Mrosek, J.; Ristow, O.; Engel, M.; Freudlsperger, C.; Freier, K.; Hoffmann, J. Multiple Sequential Free Flap Reconstructions of the Head and Neck: A Single-Center Experience. *Plast. Reconstr. Surg.* **2021**, *148*, 791e–799e. [CrossRef]
50. Vamadeva, S.V.; Henry, F.P.; Mace, A.; Clarke, P.M.; Wood, S.H.; Jallali, N. Secondary free tissue transfer in head and neck reconstruction. *J. Plast. Reconstr. Aesthet. Surg.* **2019**, *72*, 1129–1134. [CrossRef]
51. Hanasono, M.M.; Corbitt, C.A.; Yu, P.; Skoracki, R.J. Success of sequential free flaps in head and neck reconstruction. *J. Plast. Reconstr. Aesthet. Surg.* **2014**, *67*, 1186–1193. [CrossRef] [PubMed]
52. Maricevich, M.; Lin, L.O.; Liu, J.; Chang, E.I.; Hanasono, M.M. Interposition Vein Grafting in Head and Neck Free Flap Reconstruction. *Plast. Reconstr. Surg.* **2018**, *142*, 1025–1034. [CrossRef] [PubMed]
53. Di Taranto, G.; Chen, S.H.; Elia, R.; Sitpahul, N.; Chan, J.C.Y.; Losco, L.; Cigna, E.; Ribuffo, D.; Chen, H.C. Outcomes following head neck free flap reconstruction requiring interposition vein graft or vascular bridge flap. *Head Neck* **2019**, *41*, 2914–2920. [CrossRef] [PubMed]
54. Raghuram, A.C.; Manfro, G.; Teixeira, G.V.; Cernea, C.R.; Dias, F.L.; Marco, M.; Polo, R.; Abu-Ghname, A.; Maricevich, M. Use of Single Chimeric Free Flaps or Double Free Flaps for Complex Head and Neck Reconstruction. *J. Reconstr. Microsurg.* **2021**, *37*, 791–798. [CrossRef]

Disclaimer/Publisher's Note: The statements, opinions and data contained in all publications are solely those of the individual author(s) and contributor(s) and not of MDPI and/or the editor(s). MDPI and/or the editor(s) disclaim responsibility for any injury to people or property resulting from any ideas, methods, instructions or products referred to in the content.

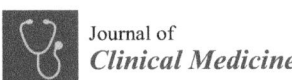

Article

Building Complex Autologous Breast Reconstruction Program: A Preliminary Experience

Min-Jeong Cho *, Christopher A. Slater, Roman J. Skoracki and Albert H. Chao

Department of Plastic and Reconstructive Surgery, The Ohio State University Wexner Medical Center, Columbus, OH 43210, USA; christopher.slater@osumc.edu (C.A.S.); roman.skoracki@osumc.edu (R.J.S.); albert.chao@osumc.edu (A.H.C.)
* Correspondence: min-jeong.cho@osumc.edu

Abstract: Autologous breast reconstruction is an increasingly popular method of reconstruction for breast cancer survivors. While deep inferior epigastric perforator (DIEP) flaps are the gold standard, not all patients are ideal candidates for DIEP flaps due to low BMI, body habitus, or previous abdominal surgery. In these patients, complex autologous breast reconstruction can be performed, but there is a limited number of programs around the world due to high technical demand. Given the increased demand and need for complex autologous flaps, it is critical to build programs to increase patient access and teach future microsurgeons. In this paper, we discuss the steps, pearls, and preliminary experience of building a complex autologous breast reconstruction program in a tertiary academic center. We performed a retrospective chart review of patients who underwent starting the year prior to the creation of our program. Since the start of our program, a total of 74 breast mounds have been reconstructed in 46 patients using 87 flaps. Over 23 months, there was a decrease in median surgical time for bilateral reconstruction by 124 min ($p = 0.03$), an increase in the number of co-surgeon cases by 66% ($p < 0.01$), and an increase in the number of complex autologous breast reconstruction by 42% ($p < 0.01$). Our study shows that a complex autologous breast reconstruction program can be successfully established using a multi-phase approach, including the development of a robust co-surgeon model. In addition, we found that a dedicated program leads to increased patient access, decreased operative time, and enhancement of trainee education.

Keywords: breast reconstruction; free flap; microsurgery; deep inferior epigastric perforator flap; profunda artery perforator flap; lumbar artery perforator flap; four-flap; complex autologous breast reconstruction; co-surgeon

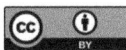

1. Introduction

Breast cancer is the most common cancer diagnosis in the United States, affecting one in eight women [1]. About 36% of breast cancer patients undergo mastectomies as a treatment, and 25% of these patients elect to have autologous-based reconstruction [2,3]. Autologous-based breast reconstruction uses a patient's own tissue, typically from the patient's abdomen, to restore the patient's whole breast after mastectomy. It offers several advantages over an implant-based reconstruction, including aesthetically pleasing, natural feeling, and long-lasting breasts with higher patient satisfaction rates [4]. Living tissue transfer using deep inferior epigastric perforator (DIEP) flaps from the abdomen is the gold standard of abdominally based autologous breast reconstruction [5]. In this procedure, the soft tissue and fat from the abdomen are transferred to the patient's chest, and microanastomosis is performed between the chest recipient vessels and the donor's vessels. Recently, there has been a significant increase in the rate of autologous breast reconstruction due to the concerns of breast implant-associated anaplastic large cell lymphoma (BIA-ALCL) in textured implants and breast implant illnesses [6–8]. These concerns led to a 112% increase in the number of autologous-based reconstructions from 2009 to 2016 [9,10].

With the increased popularity and interest in autologous-based breast reconstruction, microsurgeons developed different reconstructive techniques for patients who are not candidates for abdominally based autologous reconstruction due to previous abdominoplasty, paucity of tissue, and patient preference [11,12]. Techniques such as stacked flaps, thigh-based flaps, and trunk-based flaps have been described to expand options for autologous breast reconstruction [13]. However, these options are technically demanding procedures that require technical expertise, longer operative time, and a team of microsurgeons [14]. Despite its disadvantages, complex autologous flaps offer unique autologous options for patients who were previously denied this reconstructive option due to tissue deficiencies and underwent multiple revisionary procedures due to a lack of available microsurgeons who can perform these procedures.

Given the increased demand for autologous breast reconstruction and the growing need for complex autologous flaps, it is critical to build programs that will offer this unique option for breast cancer patients and teach future microsurgeons to ultimately increase access for patients. In this paper, we discuss the steps, pearls, and pitfalls of building a program that offers complex autologous breast reconstruction in a tertiary academic center. We will review various options for complex autologous reconstruction and phases of building the program and present preliminary data to show the successes and challenges we have faced in building a complex autologous program for breast reconstruction.

1.1. Types of Complex Autologous Breast Reconstruction

1.1.1. Surgical Techniques: DIEP Flaps

In autologous breast reconstruction, the gold standard is the deep inferior epigastric perforator (DIEP) flap, accounting for nearly 70% of autologous reconstructions [3]. This flap was first described in 1992 by Allen and Treece. In this flap, the hemiabdomen is harvested, and the deep inferior epigastric vessels, which normally supply the inferior portion of the rectus abdominus muscle, serve as its pedicle. In contrast to the transverse rectus abdominus myocutaneous (TRAM) flap, DIEP flaps spare the majority of the rectus abdominus muscle, decreasing complications at the donor site [5,15]. A reported average DIEP weight is 681 g with a range of 284 g–1504 g [16]. The average deep inferior epigastric artery is from 2 to 3 mm in diameter, with veins between 2 and 3.5 mm in diameter [5]. DIEP perforator flaps are the preferred flaps due to their low donor-site morbidity, robust vascularity, and ample volume. Yet, there are limitations to this technique, including past abdominal surgeries, inadequate abdominal fat, and poor DIEP perforators [17].

1.1.2. Surgical Techniques: APEX Flaps

The APEX (abdominal perforator exchange) flap was described to minimize the damage and dissection of the rectus abdominus muscle during the flap harvest. In the APEX flap, deep inferior epigastric vessels are harvested, but the abdominal wall structures are preserved by temporarily dividing the perforator or pedicle and reconstructing them at the end of dissection. Once outside the patient, the ligated vessels are microanastomosed [18]. This technique is recommended when more than one-third of the muscle belly or thickness could be lost, or two or more motor branches would be divided during isolation, especially in cases of lateral row perforators [18]. While this technique preserves the rectus abdominis muscle, it is very technically challenging and time-intensive to perform additional microanastomosis. Therefore, complex surgical cases like this benefit greatly from a co-surgeon model, which allows for shorter operative time [19].

1.1.3. Surgical Techniques: Double-Pedicled DIEP Flaps

Double-pedicle DIEP flaps have been described to overcome some limitations of the conventional DIEP flaps. In this technique, the entire abdomen is harvested with two pedicles to reconstruct a single breast mound [12]. Typically, patients requiring a significant amount of skin and soft tissue after radiation for unilateral breast reconstruction benefit from double-pedicled DIEP flaps or any variation in conjoined/stacked flaps [12]. Often, the cranial and caudal internal mammary vessels are recipients of the flap, but at times, it is required to use intraflap anastomoses for adequate blood flow [12,20]. This requires complex pre-surgical planning and significant technical expertise from the co-surgeons involved in the case [12,20].

1.1.4. Surgical Techniques: PAP Flaps

With advances in microsurgery, thigh-based autologous breast reconstruction options became available for patients who are not ideal candidates for abdominally based flaps. The profunda artery perforator (PAP) flap was originally used for pressure sores until its use was first described for breast reconstruction by Allen et al. in 2012 [21,22]. This flap is located on the posterior medial thigh, approximately 1 cm below the gluteal crease. The shape of the flap is long and elliptical, with an average weight of 367.4 g [21,23]. The average size of the perforator for this flap has been reported to be 1.9 mm [24]. The PAP flap has become a second choice when DIEP flaps are not an option or when a patient does not prefer the abdomen as a donor site [25]. The PAP flap can be used in various configurations, including stacked PAP flaps for unilateral breast reconstruction and four-flap procedure, which utilizes bilateral PAP and DIEP flaps for bilateral breast reconstruction [26].

1.1.5. Surgical Techniques: TUG Flaps

The transverse upper gracilis (TUG) flap is another form of thigh-based flap available to patients, first described in 1992 by Yousif et al. [27]. It varies from the PAP flap in its more anterior position, and the TUG flap involves harvesting part of the gracilis muscle. The vascular supply for a TUG flap is the medial femoral circumflex, with an average artery diameter of 1.6 mm [28]. While this flap avoids abdominal scars, the soft tissue volume can be limited. However, the advantage of the TUG flap is the high plasticity of the tissue, which is more moldable than abdominal flaps and significantly more moldable than gluteal flaps [28]. This feature makes the TUG flap ideal in cases of skin-sparing mastectomy in women with small to medium breast sizes [28].

1.1.6. Surgical Techniques: LAP Flaps

In 2003, de Weerd et al. first described the use of the lumbar artery perforator (LAP) flap for breast reconstruction. The LAP flap is supplied by the lumbar perforators at L3 and L4, where they run posterior to the psoas major muscle [29]. On average, the LAP flap has perforators with a diameter of 2.1 to 2.8 mm [30]. It is predicted that flaps as large as 21×12 cm may be harvested with flap weights reported as high as 750 g [30]. The location of the scar for a LAP flap is able to be hidden below the waistline and found to be satisfactory to patients [31]. However, the use of this flap is limited to experienced microsurgeons for several reasons. First, the flap needs to be harvested in a prone position due to its location, and the flap undergoes significant ischemia time as the patient needs to be flipped to a supine position for microanastomosis [29]. In addition, the LAP flap has a very short pedicle, which often requires the use of a vascular interposition graft to lengthen the length of the pedicle [12,29,32]. Due to the risk of prolonged ischemia times and the potential need for vascular interposition graft, the LAP flap often requires a well-orchestrated microsurgical team [33].

1.1.7. Surgical Techniques: Four-Flaps

The most complex type of autologous breast reconstruction is a four-flap procedure. This involves reconstructing a patient's breast with bilateral stacked flaps, which requires significant technical expertise. Typically, four-flap procedures are performed in patients with a lack of adequate soft tissue in one donor site to reconstruct the desired size of breast mounds [12]. The four-flap procedure is typically performed with bilateral DIEP and PAP flaps. The PAP flap is typically placed at the inframammary fold, while the DIEP flap is placed superiorly to restore the superior pole of the breast [12]. If harvesting flaps from the thigh is not an option, the LAP flap can be used in combination with the DIEP flap.

1.2. Steps of Building Complex Autologous Breast Reconstruction Program

1.2.1. Phase 1—Establishing the Co-Surgeon Model

Infrastructure

The division of Oncologic Plastic Surgery at The Ohio State University Comprehensive Cancer Center—The James—has a total of seven microsurgeons. Of these, six microsurgeons specialize in breast cancer reconstruction. In order to build a complex autologous breast reconstruction program, it is critical to build a multi-disciplinary team that specializes in the care of breast cancer reconstruction patients. We first began by introducing the co-surgeon model in which two or more microsurgeons operate simultaneously to decrease operative time and increase efficiency (Figure 1). Typically, microsurgical autologous transfer requires multiple operative steps, including the following: (1) preparation of recipient chest vessels; (2) flap elevation; (3) flap harvest; (4) microsurgical anastomosis between recipient and donor vessels under microscope; (5) inset of flaps; and (6) closure of donor sites. Given the significant number of operative steps, the co-surgeon model was introduced and has been a widely accepted practice for bilateral autologous breast reconstruction in the United States. Studies have shown that this model led to a decrease in operative time and complication, suggesting a synergistic effect [34–37].

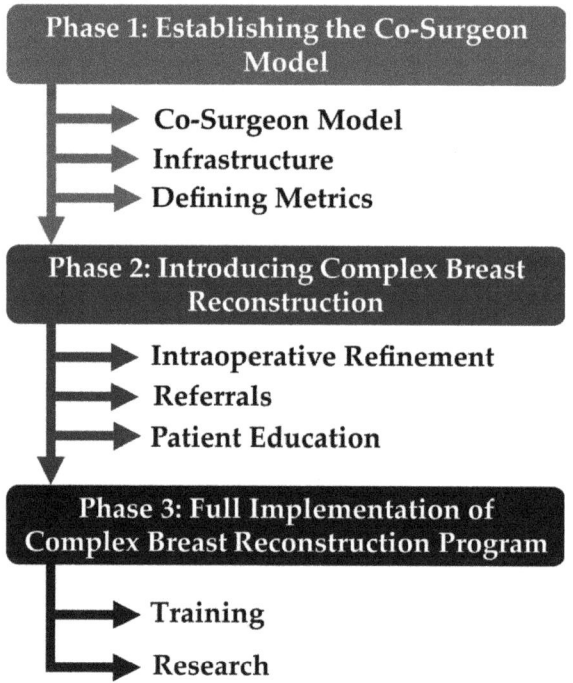

Figure 1. Roadmap of building a complex autologous breast reconstruction program.

Therefore, we started co-surgeon practice during phase 1 to create teams of efficient microsurgeons who can perform complex autologous flaps. Due to the lack of a robust co-surgeon model at The Ohio State University, we allowed 3 months for the integration of phase 1. This accounted for a few roadblocks: (1) effective scheduling of two microsurgeons; (2) preparation of the operating room team for a two-team set-up with different surgeon preferences; and (3) time period to assess the efficacy and efficiency of the model. As surgery schedulers, operating room team, anesthesia team, and trainees are not familiar with the co-surgeon model, we held multiple team conferences and education sessions to allow for an easy transition into this model. As our institution is a teaching hospital, the co-surgeon model had a team of two attending microsurgeons, one microfellow or senior resident, and one junior resident. Typically, one attending surgeon and one junior resident dissected the chest recipient vessels while the other team harvested the flaps. All patients were placed in the breast reconstruction-specific Enhanced Recovery After Surgery (ERAS) protocol, including preoperative counseling, standardized anesthetic regimen, multi-modal pain regimen, and early mobilization to achieve early recovery and decrease prolonged hospitalization [38].

Outcomes Metrics

As part of our research focus, we recorded objective metrics that could be used for identifying areas of success and areas of improvement. These factors include many items such as flap size, perforator size, ischemia time, techniques used during surgery, complication data, hospitalization data, and other factors necessary to assess our outcomes.

1.2.2. Phase 2—Introducing Complex Autologous Breast Reconstruction
Intraoperative Refinements

During phase 2, we first assessed the pitfalls and success of performing the co-surgeon model for autologous breast reconstruction. Due to scheduling conflicts, we first had pairs of microsurgeons that were matched based on their availability. However, we recognized that different microsurgeons with multiple backgrounds have different surgical preferences and approaches toward an operation. Therefore, we developed two surgical teams that consistently worked together to increase team efficiency.

Once we had two consistent microsurgical teams, we then proceeded to introduce complex autologous breast reconstruction flaps. As the operating room staff was not familiar with specific operating room set-ups of these flaps, multiple team conference was held to discuss the following: (1) PAP flaps—a frog-legged, supine position set-up with bilateral lower extremity prepping; (2) LAP flaps—multiple position changes from supine to prone to supine, prepping of different body site per position change, and set up of back table microanastomosis between the flap and interposition grafts; and (3) four-flap—prepping of both abdomen and thighs.

Referrals

Traditionally, patients who are not ideal candidates for DIEP flaps but require or desire autologous reconstruction due to radiation or patient preferences underwent latissimus dorsi flaps with implant [20,39]. As this method of reconstruction was the gold standard in patients with thin body habitus, other practitioners are not familiar with other complex autologous reconstruction options for these patients. Therefore, phase 2 was dedicated to the introduction of the complex autologous breast reconstruction program to other specialties, patients, and microsurgeons while performing these flaps in indicated patients.

We first aimed to increase internal referrals by introducing the program during grand rounds of OSU's Stefanie Spielman Comprehensive Breast Center and its affiliated hospitals. This allowed for other specialties to be familiar with the program and its referral process. In addition, we collaborated with the informational technology team to ensure that internal referral processes were in place and these referred patients were seen by the specialist teams. Subsequently, the referral processes were expanded to receive external referrals by increasing the community outreach to physicians practicing in regional cities and neighboring states. Similar to the internal referral process, grand rounds and regional conferences were utilized as the platform to share our program.

Patient Education

To increase the use of complex autologous flaps for breast reconstruction, it is important to engage patients in comprehensive patient education. Our institution has over 15 different patient education pamphlets totaling approximately 40 pages, specifically on autologous breast reconstruction. These pamphlets include many additional high-quality external resources to further educate patients.

1.2.3. Phase 3—Full Implementation of Complex Autologous Breast Reconstruction Training

Currently, our institution has one microsurgeon who was trained to perform all types of complex autologous breast reconstruction. While it is feasible to perform these types of flaps without prior training, the efficiency and efficacy of operation significantly increase with previous experience. Therefore, we are currently performing complex autologous breast reconstruction as the co-surgeon model with the pairing of experienced and non-experienced microsurgeons to increase the efficiency of the operation and to allow the partnering microsurgeon to develop an extensive understanding of nuances, pearls, and pitfalls of each complex autologous breast reconstruction.

In addition, our institution has a robust microsurgery fellowship program and plastic surgery residency program. Given that there is a limited number of institutions that specialize in complex autologous breast reconstruction, microsurgery fellows have a unique opportunity to learn and perform these procedures. Resident involvement in microsurgery is incredibly important for the education and safety of the patients [40,41]. As a team, microsurgery fellows and residents are an integral part of the complex autologous breast reconstruction program: junior residents on the recipient team and senior residents and microsurgery fellows on the flap harvest team. We plan to expand our program's impact by training individuals who will be key stakeholders in building the complex autologous breast reconstruction program nationwide.

Research

We consistently recorded objective metrics to allow for assessment, improvement, and refinement of current program performance, patient access, and trainee education. We are currently in the process of implementing the BREAST-Q to incorporate patient-reported outcomes, which may shed light on the ways to improve patient outcomes in complex autologous breast reconstruction [42,43].

2. Materials and Methods

After obtaining institutional review board approval (Institutional Review Board of The Ohio State University; #2019E0643), we performed a chart review of the electronic medical record of patients who underwent complex autologous breast reconstruction flaps from 1 September 2020 to 1 August 2023. We divided this time period into four phases: phase zero; phase one; phase two; and phase three. The first surgical case of the program occurred on 22 September 2021. Phase zero was defined by the year before the founding of the complex autologous breast reconstruction program and served as a reference year for comparisons (from 1 September 2020 to 20 September 2021). Phase one represents the time needed to establish the use of the co-surgeon model for DIEP flaps (from 22 September 2021 to 31 December 2021). Phase two and phase three are the first and second years of offering complex autologous reconstruction options (from 1 January 2022 to 31 December 2022 and from 1 January 2023 to 1 August 2023, respectively).

Retrospective chart review was conducted to collect data on patient characteristics (age, body mass index, and comorbidities), intraoperative flap data (type of flap, weight, ischemia time, procedure time, and hospital length of stay), and complications. Once the data from the chart review were collected, we utilized Excel (Microsoft 365, Redmond, WA, USA) and Prism (version 10.1.0, Boston, MA, USA) to process the data and run statistical analyses.

3. Results

In total, our program has reconstructed 74 breast mounds in 46 patients using 87 flaps (Table 1). Thirty-two patients underwent DIEP flaps, while 14 patients underwent complex autologous breast reconstruction (Table 1). Of the complex breast reconstruction patients, PAP flaps were most commonly performed, followed by LAP flaps (Table 1). Patients in the complex breast reconstruction group had lower BMI and lower rates of smokers, but the results were not statistically significant (Table 2).

Table 1. Characteristics of flaps.

	Flaps (n)	Patients (n)	Average Ischemia Time (min)	Weight (Grams)	Surgical Time (min)	Length of Stay (Days)	BMI
DIEP	57	32	73	669	523	3.7	30.2
4-Flap	16	4	76	429	719	5.0	26.8
PAP	7	4	75	310	458	3.0	28.6
LAP	5	4	144	945	613	3.5	30.2
APEX	2	2	58	549	398	3.0	29.0
Total	87	46	78	629	537	3.7	29.7

DIEP, deep inferior epigastric artery; PAP, profunda artery perforator; LAP, lumbar artery perforator; APEX, abdominal perforator exchange; BMI, body mass index.

Table 2. Clinical characteristics of the program population.

Characteristic	Overall	DIEP	Complex	p
Number of Patients	46	32	14	
Number of Flaps	87	57	30	
Number of Breast Mounds Reconstructed	74	55	19	
Age (years)	51 (25–70)	52 (25–70)	49 (33–63)	0.58
BMI	29.6 (17.5–40.9)	30.1 (17.5–39.4)	28.6 (21.2–40.9)	0.33
Bra Cup Size (Self-Reported)				
A	4.3%	6.3%	0%	
B	13%	9.4%	21.4%	
C	52.2%	59.4%	35.7%	
D	8.7%	3.1%	21.4%	
≥DD	17.4%	21.9%	7.1%	
Unknown	4.3%	0%	14.3%	
Length of Stay (days)	3.7 (2–7)	3.7 (2–7)	3.7 (3–6)	0.87
Comorbidities				
Smoking				
Never	63%	56.3%	78.6%	0.15
Current	2.2%	3.1%	0%	0.50
Former	34.8%	40.6%	21.4%	0.21
Radiation History	46.5%	51.7%	35.7%	0.48
Chemotherapy History	73.9%	78.1%	64.3%	0.33
Diabetes mellitus	4.3%	3.1%	7.1%	0.54
Hypertension	13%	18.8%	0%	0.08
ASA Physical Status	2.3 (2–3)	2.3 (2–3)	2.4 (2–3)	0.53

DIEP, deep inferior epigastric artery; BMI, body mass index; ASA, American Society of Anesthesiologists.

3.1. Demographics

There was no statistical difference between patients who received DIEP reconstruction versus complex reconstruction for age (52 yr. vs. 49 yr., $p = 0.58$), BMI (30.1 vs. 28.6, $p = 0.33$), length of stay (3.7 days vs. 3.7 days, $p = 0.87$), smoking history (43.7% vs. 21.4%, $p = 0.15$), radiation history (51.7% vs. 35.7%, $p = 0.48$), chemotherapy history (78.1% vs. 64.3%, $p = 0.33$), diabetes mellitus history (3.1% vs. 7.1%, $p = 0.51$), hypertension (18.8% vs. 0%, $p = 0.08$) and American Society of Anesthesiologist status (2.3 vs. 2.4, $p = 0.53$)

3.2. Phase Zero

During phase zero, a total of 136 breast mounds were reconstructed in 96 patients using 140 flaps. The DIEP flap accounted for nearly all of the reconstruction (98%), with a single case of four-flap and a single case of bilateral PAP flap reconstruction (Figure 2). Seventy-two percent of cases during this period were performed with a solo surgeon model (Figure 3).

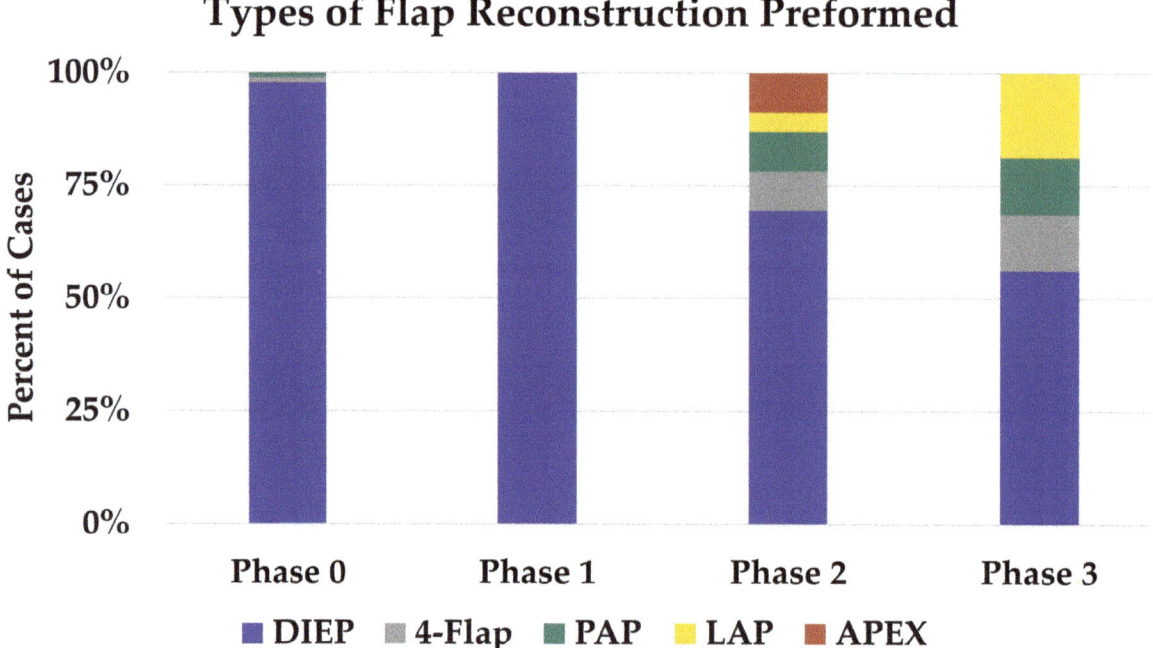

Figure 2. Trends in types of autologous breast reconstruction in our program. DIEP, deep inferior epigastric artery; PAP, profunda artery perforator; LAP, lumbar artery perforator; APEX, abdominal perforator exchange.

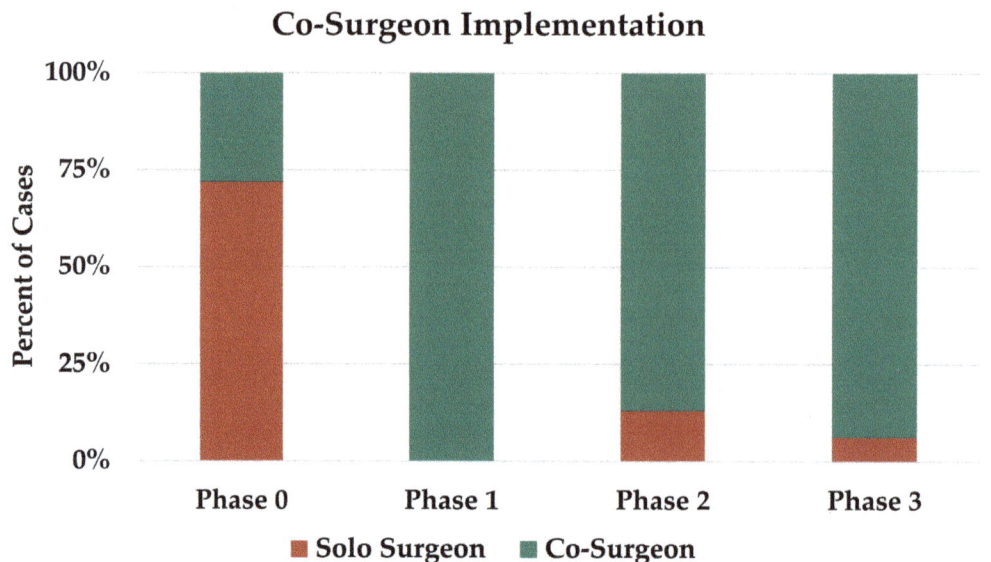

Figure 3. Trends in single and co-surgeon cases in our program.

3.3. Phase One

During phase one, focus was placed on the introduction of the co-surgeon model for DIEP flaps. In this phase, 100% of cases were performed using the co-surgeon model, which lasted from 22 September 2021 to 31 December 2021 (Figure 1). This phase was dedicated to maximizing efficiency and building a team, and all reconstructions in this time period were DIEP flaps (Figure 3). The average operative time for DIEP flaps decreased by 122 min from an average of 638 min in phase zero ($p = 0.05$).

3.4. Phase Two

In phase two, we focused on expanding the use of complex autologous flaps. During this phase, the proportion of complex autologous flaps increased from 0% to 30% of cases (Figure 3). During this period, two four-flaps, two PAP flaps, one LAP flap, and two APEX flaps were performed (Figure 3).

3.5. Phase Three

As the program continued to expand, we reached phase three, the full implementation of complex autologous breast reconstruction, 15 months after founding the program. During phase three, we continued the co-surgeon model, except when unilateral non-complex autologous breast reconstruction was performed (6%). Given the increased familiarity with preoperative planning, intraoperative set-up, and postoperative care, we increased the number and complexity of the flaps performed. During this period, complex reconstruction accounted for 44% of cases (two four-flaps, two PAP flaps, and three LAP flaps).

3.6. Program Effect on Surgical Times

Overall, there was a decrease in median surgical time for bilateral reconstruction of 124 min (652 min vs. 528 min, $p = 0.03$) after the creation of the program. The average surgical time decreased for bilateral co-surgeon (68 min, $p = 0.05$) and bilateral DIEP reconstruction (77 min, $p = 0.01$). After the start of the program, there has been an increase in co-surgeon unilateral breast reconstruction due to the rise in the complexity of unilateral reconstruction, such as stacked PAP flaps and LAP flaps. For stacked PAP flap cases, two PAP flaps were harvested to create one breast mound. Both flaps are microanastomosed to the internal mammary vessels using the anterograde and retrograde vessels. Due to the increase in the technical demand for these flaps, co-surgeon unilateral complex reconstruction took, on average, 112 min longer than co-surgeon unilateral DIEP reconstruction ($p = 0.016$). For overall complex reconstruction, there was a decrease of 184 min in the median operation time and 134 min in the mean. However, there were only two complex reconstructions in our control period prior to program creation, so statistical significance was not noted ($p = 0.15$).

3.7. Complications

There was no statistically significant difference in the overall complication rate for the DIEP flaps vs. complex flaps (18% vs. 17%, $p = 0.92$) (Table 3). The most common complication was take-backs (seven flaps, 8%) (Table 3); the most common cause of take-backs was due to venous congestion (three flaps). However, our salvage rate was 100% during the hospitalization, and there was one single DIEP flap failure on postoperative day 15 due to a fall onto the flap. For four-flap reconstruction, the most common complications were take-backs occurring twice, hematoma occurring once, and pneumonia occurring in one patient (Table 3). We did not encounter any complications with PAP flaps and APEX flaps. Lumbar artery perforator flaps had one case of breast infection and one case of seroma (Table 3). The Clavien–Dindo classification for the complications showed that the majority of complications required surgical intervention under general anesthesia. Ninety percent (nine patients) of the 3b complications were due to take-backs, with 10% (1 patient) due to flap failure from vessel avulsion. We have no type 1, 4, or 5 complications. The type 2 complication was medication given for an infection (Table 4).

Table 3. Characteristics of complications.

	Infection (%)	Take-Back (%)	Seroma (%)	Hematoma (%)	Wound Dehiscence (%)	Fat Necrosis (%)	Flap Failure (%)	Deep Vein Thrombosis (%)
DIEP	0	9	0	2	2	2	2	3
4-Flap	0	13	0	6	0	0	0	0
PAP	0	0	0	0	0	0	0	0
LAP	20	0	20	0	0	0	0	0
APEX	0	0	0	0	0	0	0	0
Overall	1	8	1	2	1	1	1	2

DIEP, deep inferior epigastric artery; PAP, profunda artery perforator; LAP, lumbar artery perforator; APEX, abdominal perforator exchange.

Table 4. Clavien–Dindo classification of complications.

	0 (n)	1 (n)	2 (n)	3a (n)	3b (n)	4 (n)	5 (n)
DIEP	24	0	1	0	7	0	0
4-Flap	1	0	0	0	3	0	0
PAP	4	0	0	0	0	0	0
LAP	2	0	0	2	0	0	0
APEX	2	0	0	0	0	0	0
Overall	33	0	1	2	10	0	0

DIEP, deep inferior epigastric artery; PAP, profunda artery perforator; LAP, lumbar artery perforator; APEX, abdominal perforator exchange.

4. Discussion

Autologous breast reconstruction is the gold standard for providing natural, long-lasting breast reconstruction that often leads to higher patient satisfaction and aesthetic outcomes [4]. While the DEIP flap is the most commonly performed flap for autologous breast reconstruction, many patients are not ideal candidates for DIEP flaps due to low BMI, previous abdominoplasty, or the need for additional soft tissue [12,13]. Traditionally, these patients would undergo a combined autologous breast reconstruction such as latissimus dorsi flap and implant. However, this procedure still uses a prosthetic, which carries the risk of implant failure, infection, capsular contracture, and the need for implant exchange. Therefore, plastic surgeons have developed multiple novel techniques, such as multiple free flaps, using stacked flaps from non-abdomen donor sites. Despite the potentially higher patient satisfaction and aesthetic outcomes from complex autologous breast reconstruction, there is a limited number of centers offering this type of reconstruction due to the technically demanding nature of these procedures, longer operative time, and need for multiple microsurgeons [14]. With the increased concerns over implants due to breast implant-associated anaplastic large cell lymphoma, there has been a growing need for autologous breast reconstruction, and it is critical to build a center with a complex autologous breast reconstruction program.

Our preliminary experience of implementing a complex autologous breast reconstruction program shows that this program can be successfully established using a multi-phase approach. Since the start of our program, a total of 74 breast mounds have been reconstructed in 46 patients using 87 flaps. Over 23 months, there was a decrease in median surgical time for bilateral reconstruction by 124 min ($p = 0.03$), an increase in the number of co-surgeon cases by 66% ($p < 0.01$), and an increase in the number of complex autologous breast reconstruction by 42% ($p < 0.01$). The co-surgeon model was instrumental to the success of building this program as it allowed microsurgeons to adapt to new techniques and build team efficiency [14,19,35]. Two co-surgeon teams consisted of one junior microsurgeon experienced with complex flap breast reconstruction and one senior microsurgeon with at least 5 years of practice with no prior experience. By allowing the combination of years of technical excellence and familiarity with complex flaps, we were able to perform

30 complex flaps in 14 patients during 23 months of the program. While our average operative time of complex flaps (568 min) is higher than the published range of 520.7 to 610.3 min, we believe that operative time will continue to improve as microsurgeons, operating room staff, and trainees gain more experience [6,44].

Despite the infancy of our program, we have performed a wide range of complex autologous breast reconstructions, including unilateral stacked PAP flaps, bilateral PAP flaps, LAP flaps, four flaps using bilateral DIEP/PAP flaps, four flaps using bilateral DIEP/LAP flaps, and APEX flaps. The range of operative time was from 398 to 719 min, and the range of hospitalization was from 3 to 5 days. The most common complication in complex autologous breast reconstruction was take-back (7% vs. 8% in DIEP flaps). However, this only occurred in four-flap patients, which was most likely due to increased complexity and having flaps buried in stacked flaps. To maximize the aesthetic appearance of the reconstructed breasts, we frequently bury flaps in stacked flap breast reconstruction. While other monitoring mechanisms, such as implantable Doppler, are placed, it is challenging to fully assess the flap when the flap cannot be visualized [45]. Therefore, we have a low threshold for taking our complex flaps back to the operating room for exploration and potential flap salvage as needed. The majority of our flap take-backs were due to venous congestion secondary to pedicle positioning. To allow for stacked flap configuration, flap pedicles are placed in a specific configuration (anterograde anastomosis of a caudally placed flap and retrograde anastomosis of a cranially placed flap using internal mammary vessels or thoracodorsal vessels) within a breast pocket [46]. Given that flap pedicles must cross, it is critical to place the pedicles in an orientation that the pedicles will not kink or compress. Similarly, Haddock et al. found that stacked flap reconstruction has a higher rate of flap take-back but similar rates of flap failure rate between single and stacked flap breast reconstruction [6]. In our experience, all complex flaps were salvaged despite the higher flap take-back rate.

In addition, our program was able to successfully increase the number of complex flaps while maintaining a similar complication profile as single-flap breast reconstruction. Despite the increased number of donor sites in patients undergoing complex autologous breast reconstruction, the rate of donor-site complications was similar between DIEP and complex flaps except for the rate of seroma in LAP patients (one out of five donor sites). Studies have shown that the rate of seroma was higher than in traditional donor sites, and we have begun to perform more aggressive donor site closure and use of compression to decrease the rate of seroma [31]. Interestingly, our length of stay in complex flaps stayed similar to patients undergoing DIEP flaps except for the four-flap patients. As these patients stayed an average of 1 to 2 days longer than other complex flaps, we believe that this finding is secondary to the pain and difficulty with mobilization due to multiple-donor sites. In addition, the length of operative time is longer in these patients, and studies showed that there is a 27% increase in the risk of a postoperative complication for every additional hour of operative time in bilateral autologous breast reconstruction [35]. Therefore, one of our goals is to decrease the operative time in four-flap patients by 60 min by the end of phase 3.

Future directions to this program include (1) expanding the co-surgeon model, (2) increasing patient access through dedicated training, and (3) refining the program with our research findings. Currently, the main co-surgeon model that we use involves both surgeons being present for the entirety of reconstruction. However, this type of scheduling requires the co-surgeon to forego an entire operative day when they could have performed additional operative cases. As our operative experience grows and the program becomes busier, we plan to transition our co-surgeon model to a model when co-surgeons assist in two staggered cases during the key portion of the case. Studies have shown that this model can be safely performed while decreasing the operative time, length of stay, and wound complications [14,35]. In this advanced co-surgeon model, we can decrease the average wait time for the operation and increase patient access. We anticipate that with the addition of new microsurgeons who have significant training in performing complex autologous breast reconstruction, we will be able to implement the advanced co-surgeon model.

Secondly, we will focus our efforts on increasing patient access through dedicated training of microsurgery fellows. For our program, the key factors of successful development included a high-volume center, experienced microsurgeons, multi-disciplinary collaboration, and a microsurgeon who is well-experienced in performing complex autologous breast reconstruction. We believe that having one microsurgeon who is well-versed with these types of procedures leads to multi-magnitude effects on patient care by greatly expanding breast reconstruction options to patients with an insufficient single-donor site, irradiated patients with significant pliable skin requirement, and patients with failed implant-based breast reconstruction to obtain a natural, ptotic breast. While Bodin et al. showed that a minimum of 50 cases are needed to be proficient in DIEP flaps, we believe that it would take a lesser number of flaps to become proficient in complex autologous breast reconstruction as the principle of perforator dissection and flap harvest does not change [47,48]. Therefore, we believe that one year of the microsurgery fellowship program would be sufficient to train and increase proficiency in microsurgery fellows. As evident from our program, it is critical to increase the number of these microsurgeons who can team up with their partners to sustain continued relationships with our center and educate future microsurgeons, which will ultimately increase patient access nationwide.

Lastly, we believe that outcome research is critical to the continued development and refinement of the program. Since the beginning of our program, we have instituted multiple protocols based on outcome metrics. We collected various perioperative metrics, including the following: (1) preoperative—referral patterns, patient characteristics, preoperative planning using computed tomography angiography (CTA), co-surgeon scheduling, and team efficiency; (2) intraoperative—operative time, intraoperative set-up time, co-surgeon involvement, and trainee participation; and (3) postoperative—flap monitoring, nursing staff training, and specific postoperative protocols. During the first three phases, we first focused our efforts on maximizing preoperative and intraoperative metrics to minimize complications. We have incorporated preoperative CTA for preoperative planning, intraoperative indocyanine green (ICG) angiography to evaluate the flap perfusion, use of multi-phasic bovie cautery, coordinated position change protocol, and development of dedicated flap recipient/harvest teams [20,49].

With these refinements, we were able to further decrease operative time and increase our flap success rate. However, we have noticed increased challenges in flap monitoring protocol due to the variations in the nursing staff. In contrast to a dedicated operative team and outpatient nursing staff, inpatient nursing team members change frequently, and not all members are experienced with additional flap monitoring devices such as implantable Doppler or pulse oximetry devices. Therefore, we plan to hold regular in-services discussing our program and modify our protocols as needed.

Limitations of our study include the small size of our study population. The sample size for statistical analysis is limited by the infancy of our program (<2 years of complex reconstruction) and by the fact that complex reconstruction is only suitable for certain patients. For example, we were not able to statistically analyze specific complication rates for each flap type due to the rarity of complications and small numbers of each type of complex reconstruction. Prospective data collection and expansion of our surgical team will allow us to overcome these limitations in the future.

5. Conclusions

Despite the growing need for autologous breast reconstruction using complex flaps, it has been challenging to increase the number of centers that provide these unique options to patients due to technical demand and multilevel collaboration. In this study, we have found that a complex autologous breast reconstruction program can be successfully established using a multi-phase approach, including the development of a robust co-surgeon model, and a dedicated program leads to increased patient access, decreased operative time, decreased length of stay, and enhancement of trainee education. We hope that the pearls, lessons, and challenges that we have faced will serve as a useful guide to those who wish to incorporate this program as a part of their practice.

Author Contributions: Conceptualization, M.-J.C., C.A.S., R.J.S. and A.H.C.; methodology, M.-J.C., C.A.S., R.J.S. and A.H.C.; software, M.-J.C. and C.A.S.; validation, M.-J.C. and C.A.S.; formal analysis, M.-J.C. and C.A.S.; investigation, M.-J.C. and C.A.S.; resources, M.-J.C., C.A.S., R.J.S. and A.H.C.; data curation, M.-J.C., C.A.S., R.J.S. and A.H.C.; writing—original draft preparation, M.-J.C. and C.A.S.; writing—review and editing, M.-J.C., C.A.S., R.J.S. and A.H.C.; visualization, M.-J.C. and C.A.S.; supervision, M.-J.C., R.J.S. and A.H.C.; project administration, M.-J.C., R.J.S. and A.H.C. All authors have read and agreed to the published version of the manuscript.

Funding: This research received no external funding.

Institutional Review Board Statement: This study was conducted in accordance with the Declaration of Helsinki and approved by the Institutional Review Board of The Ohio State University (#2019E0643; date of approval, 2 February 2023).

Informed Consent Statement: Informed consent was obtained from all subjects involved in this study.

Data Availability Statement: The data presented in this study are available on request from the corresponding author. The corresponding author will ensure that individual privacy and IRB compliance are not compromised during the transfer of datasets.

Conflicts of Interest: The authors declare no conflict of interest.

References

1. Common Cancer Sites—Cancer Stat Facts. 2023. Available online: https://seer.cancer.gov/statfacts/html/common.html (accessed on 5 August 2023).
2. Kummerow, K.L.; Du, L.; Penson, D.F.; Shyr, Y.; Hooks, M.A. Nationwide Trends in Mastectomy for Early-Stage Breast Cancer. *JAMA Surg.* **2015**, *150*, 9–16. [CrossRef] [PubMed]
3. Plastic Surgery Statistics. Available online: https://www.plasticsurgery.org/news/plastic-surgery-statistics (accessed on 5 August 2023).
4. Kroll, S.S.; Baldwin, B. A comparison of outcomes using three different methods of breast reconstruction. *Plast. Reconstr. Surg.* **1992**, *90*, 455–462. [CrossRef]
5. Granzow, J.W.; Levine, J.L.; Chiu, E.S.; Allen, R.J. Breast reconstruction with the deep inferior epigastric perforator flap: History and an update on current technique. *J. Plast. Reconstr. Aesthetic Surg. JPRAS* **2006**, *59*, 571–579. [CrossRef]
6. Haddock, N.T.; Cho, M.-J.; Teotia, S.S. Comparative Analysis of Single versus Stacked Free Flap Breast Reconstruction: A Single-Center Experience. *Plast. Reconstr. Surg.* **2019**, *144*, 369e–377e. [CrossRef]
7. Parham, C.S.; Hanson, S.E.; Butler, C.E.; Calobrace, M.B.; Hollrah, R.; Macgregor, T.; Clemens, M.W. Advising patients about breast implant associated anaplastic large cell lymphoma. *Gland Surg.* **2021**, *10*, 417–429. [CrossRef]
8. Pelc, Z.; Skórzewska, M.; Kurylcio, A.; Olko, P.; Dryka, J.; Machowiec, P.; Maksymowicz, M.; Rawicz-Pruszyński, K.; Polkowski, W. Current Challenges in Breast Implantation. *Medicina* **2021**, *57*, 1214. [CrossRef] [PubMed]
9. Lee, B.T.; Agarwal, J.P.; Ascherman, J.A.; Caterson, S.A.; Gray, D.D.; Hollenbeck, S.T.; Khan, S.A.; Loeding, L.D.; Mahabir, R.C.; Miller, A.S.; et al. Evidence-Based Clinical Practice Guideline: Autologous Breast Reconstruction with DIEP or Pedicled TRAM Abdominal Flaps. *Plast. Reconstr. Surg.* **2017**, *140*, 651e–664e. [CrossRef] [PubMed]
10. Masoomi, H.; Hanson, S.E.; Clemens, M.W.; Mericli, A.F. Autologous Breast Reconstruction Trends in the United States: Using the Nationwide Inpatient Sample Database. *Ann. Plast. Surg.* **2021**, *87*, 242–247. [CrossRef]
11. Reyna, C.; Lee, M.C. Breast cancer in young women: Special considerations in multidisciplinary care. *J. Multidiscip. Healthc.* **2014**, *7*, 419–429. [CrossRef]
12. Haddock, N.T.; Teotia, S.S. Modern Approaches to Alternative Flap-Based Breast Reconstruction: Stacked Flaps. *Clin. Plast. Surg.* **2023**, *50*, 325–335. [CrossRef]
13. Myers, P.L.; Nelson, J.A.; Allen, R.J., Jr. Alternative flaps in autologous breast reconstruction. *Gland Surg.* **2021**, *10*, 444–459. [CrossRef]
14. Bauermeister, A.J.; Zuriarrain, A.; Newman, M.; Earle, S.A.; Medina, M.A., 3rd. Impact of Continuous Two-Team Approach in Autologous Breast Reconstruction. *J. Reconstr. Microsurg.* **2017**, *33*, 298–304. [CrossRef] [PubMed]
15. Cho, M.-J.; Teotia, S.S.; Haddock, N.T. Predictors, Classification, and Management of Umbilical Complications in DIEP Flap Breast Reconstruction. *Plast. Reconstr. Surg.* **2017**, *140*, 11–18. [CrossRef]
16. Woo, K.-J.; Mun, G.-H. Estimation of DIEP flap weight for breast reconstruction by the pinch test. *Microsurgery* **2017**, *37*, 786–792. [CrossRef]
17. Haddock, N.T.; Cho, M.-J.; Gassman, A.; Teotia, S.S. Stacked Profunda Artery Perforator Flap for Breast Reconstruction in Failed or Unavailable Deep Inferior Epigastric Perforator Flap. *Plast. Reconstr. Surg.* **2019**, *143*, 488e–494e. [CrossRef] [PubMed]

18. Zoccali, G.; Farhadi, J. Abdominal perforator exchange flap (APEX): A classification of pedicle rearrangements. *Microsurgery* **2021**, *41*, 607–614. [CrossRef]
19. Canizares, O.; Mayo, J.; Soto, E.; Allen, R.J.; Sadeghi, A. Optimizing Efficiency in Deep Inferior Epigastric Perforator Flap Breast Reconstruction. *Ann. Plast. Surg.* **2015**, *75*, 186–192. [CrossRef]
20. Cho, M.-J.; Haddock, N.T.; Teotia, S.S. Clinical Decision Making Using CTA in Conjoined, Bipedicled DIEP and SIEA for Unilateral Breast Reconstruction. *J. Reconstr. Microsurg.* **2020**, *36*, 241–246. [CrossRef]
21. Allen, R.J.; Haddock, N.T.; Ahn, C.Y.; Sadeghi, A. Breast reconstruction with the profunda artery perforator flap. *Plast. Reconstr. Surg.* **2012**, *129*, 16e–23e. [CrossRef]
22. Haddock, N.T.; Gassman, A.; Cho, M.-J.; Teotia, S.S. 101 Consecutive Profunda Artery Perforator Flaps in Breast Reconstruction: Lessons Learned with Our Early Experience. *Plast. Reconstr. Surg.* **2017**, *140*, 229–239. [CrossRef] [PubMed]
23. Allen, R.J.; Lee, Z.-H.; Mayo, J.L.; Levine, J.; Ahn, C.; Allen, R.J. The Profunda Artery Perforator Flap Experience for Breast Reconstruction. *Plast. Reconstr. Surg.* **2016**, *138*, 968–975. [CrossRef] [PubMed]
24. Haddock, N.T.; Greaney, P.; Otterburn, D.; Levine, S.; Allen, R.J. Predicting perforator location on preoperative imaging for the profunda artery perforator flap. *Microsurgery* **2012**, *32*, 507–511. [CrossRef] [PubMed]
25. Cho, M.-J.; Teotia, S.S.; Haddock, N.T. Classification and Management of Donor-Site Wound Complications in the Profunda Artery Perforator Flap for Breast Reconstruction. *J. Reconstr. Microsurg.* **2020**, *36*, 110–115. [CrossRef]
26. Haddock, N.T.; Suszynski, T.M.; Teotia, S.S. Consecutive Bilateral Breast Reconstruction Using Stacked Abdominally Based and Posterior Thigh Free Flaps. *Plast. Reconstr. Surg.* **2021**, *147*, 294–303. [CrossRef] [PubMed]
27. Buchel, E.W.; Dalke, K.R.; Hayakawa, T.E. The transverse upper gracilis flap: Efficiencies and design tips. *Can. J. Plast. Surg.* **2013**, *21*, 162–166. [CrossRef]
28. Arnez, Z.M.; Pogorelec, D.; Planinsek, F.; Ahcan, U. Breast reconstruction by the free transverse gracilis (TUG) flap. *Br. J. Plast. Surg.* **2004**, *57*, 20–26. [CrossRef]
29. Stillaert, F.B.J.L.; Opsomer, D.; Blondeel, P.N.; Van Landuyt, K. The Lumbar Artery Perforator Flap in Breast Reconstruction. *Plast. Reconstr. Surg.* **2023**, *151*, 41–44. [CrossRef]
30. Vonu, P.M.; Chopan, M.; Sayadi, L.; Chim, H.W.; Leyngold, M. Lumbar Artery Perforator Flaps: A Systematic Review of Free Tissue Transfers and Anatomical Characteristics. *Ann. Plast. Surg.* **2022**, *89*, 465–471. [CrossRef]
31. Opsomer, D.; Vyncke, T.; Ryx, M.; Van Landuyt, K.; Blondeel, P.; Stillaert, F. Donor Site Morbidity after Lumbar Artery Perforator Flap Breast Reconstruction. *J. Reconstr. Microsurg.* **2022**, *38*, 129–136. [CrossRef]
32. Cho, M.-J.; Haddock, N.T.; Teotia, S.S. Harvesting Composite Arterial and Vein Grafts from Deep Inferior Epigastric Artery and Vein: A Safe Five-Step Method of Preparation. *Plast. Reconstr. Surg.* **2022**, *149*, 195e–197e. [CrossRef]
33. Haddock, N.T.; Teotia, S.S. Lumbar Artery Perforator Flap: Initial Experience with Simultaneous Bilateral Flaps for Breast Reconstruction. *Plast. Reconstr. Surg. Glob. Open* **2020**, *8*, e2800. [CrossRef] [PubMed]
34. Mericli, A.F.; Chu, C.K.; Sisk, G.C.; Largo, R.D.; Schaverien, M.V.; Liu, J.; Villa, M.T.; Garvey, P.B. Microvascular Breast Reconstruction in the Era of Value-Based Care: Use of a Cosurgeon Is Associated with Reduced Costs, Improved Outcomes, and Added Value. *Plast. Reconstr. Surg.* **2022**, *149*, 338–348. [CrossRef]
35. Razdan, S.N.; Panchal, H.J.; Hespe, G.E.; Disa, J.J.; McCarthy, C.M.; Allen, R.J., Jr.; Dayan, J.H.; Pusic, A.; Mehrara, B.; Cordeiro, P.G.; et al. The Impact of the Cosurgeon Model on Bilateral Autologous Breast Reconstruction. *J. Reconstr. Microsurg.* **2017**, *33*, 624–629. [CrossRef]
36. Contag, S.P.; Golub, J.S.; Teknos, T.N.; Nussenbaum, B.; Stack, B.C.; Arnold, D.J.; Johns, M.M. Professional Burnout Among Microvascular and Reconstructive Free-Flap Head and Neck Surgeons in the United States. *Arch. Otolaryngol.—Head Neck Surg.* **2010**, *136*, 950–956. [CrossRef] [PubMed]
37. Nguyen, P.D.; Herrera, F.A.; Roostaeian, J.; Da Lio, A.L.; Crisera, C.A.; Festekjian, J.H. Career satisfaction and burnout in the reconstructive microsurgeon in the United States. *Microsurgery* **2015**, *35*, 1–5. [CrossRef]
38. Cho, M.-J.; Garza, R.; Teotia, S.S.; Haddock, N.T. Utility of ERAS Pathway in Nonabdominal-Based Microsurgical Breast Reconstruction: Efficacy in PAP Flap Reconstruction? *J. Reconstr. Microsurg.* **2022**, *38*, 371–377. [CrossRef]
39. Mushin, O.P.; Myers, P.L.; Langstein, H.N. Indications and Controversies for Complete and Implant-Enhanced Latissimus Dorsi Breast Reconstructions. *Clin. Plast. Surg.* **2018**, *45*, 75–81. [CrossRef]
40. Albornoz, C.R.; Cordeiro, P.G.; Hishon, L.; Mehrara, B.J.; Pusic, A.L.; McCarthy, C.M.; Disa, J.J.; Matros, E. A nationwide analysis of the relationship between hospital volume and outcome for autologous breast reconstruction. *Plast. Reconstr. Surg.* **2013**, *132*, 192e–200e. [CrossRef] [PubMed]
41. Cho, M.J.; Halani, S.H.; Davis, J.; Zhang, A.Y. Achieving balance between resident autonomy and patient safety: Analysis of resident-led microvascular reconstruction outcomes at a microsurgical training center with an established microsurgical training pathway. *J. Plast. Reconstr. Aesthetic Surg.* **2020**, *73*, 118–125. [CrossRef]
42. Spoer, D.L.; Kiene, J.M.; Dekker, P.K.; Huffman, S.S.; Kim, K.G.; Abadeer, A.I.; Fan, K.L. A Systematic Review of Artificial Intelligence Applications in Plastic Surgery: Looking to the Future. *Plast. Reconstr. Surg. Glob. Open* **2022**, *10*, e4608. [CrossRef]
43. Liu, L.Q.; Branford, O.A.; Mehigan, S. BREAST-Q Measurement of the Patient Perspective in Oncoplastic Breast Surgery: A Systematic Review. *Plast. Reconstr. Surg. Glob. Open* **2018**, *6*, e1904. [CrossRef] [PubMed]
44. Haddock, N.T.; Teotia, S.S. Efficient DIEP Flap: Bilateral Breast Reconstruction in Less Than Four Hours. *Plast. Reconstr. Surg. Glob. Open* **2021**, *9*, e3801. [CrossRef]

45. Dunklebarger, M.F.; McCrary, H.; King, B.; Carpenter, P.; Buchmann, L.; Hunt, J.; Cannon, R. Success of Implantable Doppler Probes for Monitoring Buried Free Flaps. *Otolaryngol. Head Neck Surg.* **2022**, *167*, 452–456. [CrossRef] [PubMed]
46. Teotia, S.S.; Cho, M.-J.; Haddock, N.T. Salvaging Breast Reconstruction: Profunda Artery Perforator Flaps Using Thoracodorsal Vessels. *Plast. Reconstr. Surg. Glob. Open* **2018**, *6*, e1837. [CrossRef]
47. Bodin, F.; Dissaux, C.; Lutz, J.C.; Hendriks, S.; Fiquet, C.; Bruant-Rodier, C. The DIEP flap breast reconstruction: Starting from scratch in a university hospital. *Ann. Chir. Plast. Esthet.* **2015**, *60*, 171–178. [CrossRef]
48. Varnava, C.; Wiebringhaus, P.; Hirsch, T.; Dermietzel, A.; Kueckelhaus, M. Breast Reconstruction with DIEP Flap: The Learning Curve at a Breast Reconstruction Center and a Single-Surgeon Study. *J. Clin. Med.* **2023**, *12*, 2894. [CrossRef] [PubMed]
49. Johnson, A.C.; Colakoglu, S.; Chong, T.W.; Mathes, D.W. Indocyanine Green Angiography in Breast Reconstruction: Utility, Limitations, and Search for Standardization. *Plast. Reconstr. Surg. Glob. Open* **2020**, *8*, e2694. [CrossRef] [PubMed]

Disclaimer/Publisher's Note: The statements, opinions and data contained in all publications are solely those of the individual author(s) and contributor(s) and not of MDPI and/or the editor(s). MDPI and/or the editor(s) disclaim responsibility for any injury to people or property resulting from any ideas, methods, instructions or products referred to in the content.

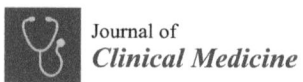 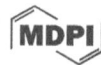

Article

Anterolateral Thigh Chimeric Flap: An Alternative Reconstructive Option to Free Flaps for Large Soft Tissue Defects

Yoon Jae Lee [1], Junnyeon Kim [2], Chae Rim Lee [2], Jun Hyeok Kim [1], Deuk Young Oh [2], Young Joon Jun [2] and Suk-Ho Moon [2,*]

[1] Department of Plastic and Reconstructive Surgery, Yeouido St. Mary's Hospital, College of Medicine, The Catholic University of Korea, Seoul 07345, Republic of Korea; yoonjae@catholic.ac.kr (Y.J.L.); hyeoggy@gmail.com (J.H.K.)

[2] Department of Plastic and Reconstructive Surgery, Seoul St. Mary's Hospital, College of Medicine, The Catholic University of Korea, Seoul 06591, Republic of Korea; sweety4512@naver.com (J.K.); chaerim.lee@gmail.com (C.R.L.); ohdeuk1234@hanmail.net (D.Y.O.); joony@catholic.ac.kr (Y.J.J.)

* Correspondence: nasuko@catholic.ac.kr

Abstract: The anterolateral thigh (ALT) skin flap provides abundant, thin, pliable skin coverage with adequate pedicle length and calibre, and tolerable donor site morbidity. However, coverage of relatively large defects using the ALT flap alone is limited. We present our experience of using the ALT flap coupled with the vastus lateralis (VL) flap supplied by the same pedicle for large defect reconstruction. Between 2016 and 2020, ten patients with extensive lower-extremity or trunk defects were treated using the ALT/VL chimeric flap. The ALT portion was used to cover the cutaneous and joint defect while the VL part was used to resurface remnant defects, and a skin graft was performed. All flaps were based on the common descending pedicle, and branches to separate the components were individually dissected. All defects were successfully reconstructed using the ALT/VL chimeric flap. No surgery-related acute complications were observed, and the patients had no clinical issues with ambulation or running activities during the long-term follow-up period. With the separate components supplied by a common vascular pedicle, the ALT/VL chimeric flap allows us to reconstruct extensive defects with joint involvement or posterior trunk lesions. Thus, the ALT/VL chimeric flap may be a suitable alternative for extensive tissue defect reconstruction.

Keywords: perforator flap; reconstructive surgical procedures; anteromedial thigh flap; vastus lateralis; microsurgery

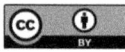

1. Introduction

An extensive resection of complex traumatic wounds or tumours often causes large soft tissue defects [1–3]. A one-stage reconstruction of large soft tissue defects is imperative to restore function and achieve aesthetic results.

Conventional reconstructive methods often rely on the use of free flaps, such as the latissimus dorsi (LD) flap and transverse rectus abdominis muscle (TRAM) flap, which have served as foundational techniques for addressing large soft tissue defects [4–8]. The LD flap, a reliable option, provides substantial tissue coverage but is associated with post-operative seroma formation and potential functional limitations in the arm [6]. On the other hand, the TRAM flap is limited to patients without a history of abdominal surgery or liposuction [9]. The need for a complete defect coverage may necessitate multiple free flap transfers, introducing increased complexity and associated risks [10,11].

Various muscle flaps, such as the gracilis flap, rectus abdominis flap, and gluteus maximus flap can be used in soft tissue reconstruction [12]. These flaps offer a generous volume of tissue for coverage and can be especially useful in cases where muscle function preservation is not a primary concern. Other perforator flaps, such as the deep inferior epigastric perforator (DIEP) flap and superior gluteal artery perforator (SGAP) flap, minimize muscle sacrifice while providing a reliable source of well-vascularized tissue. Local flaps, including rotational, advancement, and island flaps, are valuable options for smaller soft tissue defects [12,13]. Tissue expansion involves the gradual stretching of the existing skin to create additional tissue. It is useful for patients with limited donor sites and has been successfully employed in breast reconstruction and scar revision. In situations where an autologous tissue is not available or suitable, allografts or xenografts can be used for wound coverage. These options are often applied in cases of extensive burns or non-healing wounds [14–16].

The anterolateral thigh (ALT) flap has several beneficial characteristics that make it a favourable donor site for soft-tissue reconstruction of various parts of the body. These preferable characteristics include large amounts of thin, pliable skin coverage, a long vascular pedicle, convenient pedicle calibre, and minimal donor site morbidity [17–20].

However, there are some limitations in using the ALT flap alone for large defects. As advances in microsurgery have led to the development of various chimeric pattern flaps, we propose a chimeric perforator flap design in which the ALT perforator flap and vastus lateralis (VL) chimeric muscle flap are microsurgically constructed as chimeric perforator flaps to overcome the limitations of using an ALT flap alone. In addition, in the case of perforation injury during harvesting for the ALT flap, the VL muscle flap can be used as an alternative.

Although the ALT/VL muscle chimeric flap has been used to reconstruct extensive hand and neck injuries [21], studies regarding the use of this flap in the reconstruction of large trunk and lower extremity defects are limited.

In this case series, we present our experience with the ALT/VL muscle chimeric flap based on perforators from the descending branch of the lateral circumflex vessels in the reconstruction of large defects.

2. Patients and Methods

Ten patients who underwent an ALT/VL chimeric free flap in extensive lower extremity or trunk lesions—from January 2016 to December 2020—were analysed.

Operative Technique

With a hand-held Doppler, mapping of the ALT perforator(s) was routinely performed before flap elevation. The operation was performed under general anaesthesia with the patients in the supine position. The ALT perforator axis—the line connecting the lateral border of the patella and anterior superior iliac spine (ASIS)—was drawn, and based on this axis, the locations of the perforator were identified using the hand-held Doppler. To design the skin island, a template of the defect was drawn, and the perforators were included in the flap design. A pinch test was used to evaluate the feasibility of primary closure at the donor site. The flap was elevated starting from the medial border. An incision was made into the deep fascia, and the intermuscular septum was identified. After a blunt dissection of the space between the rectus femoris muscle and the VL muscle using the fingers, the descending branch of the lateral circumflex artery (LCFA) was located. After confirming the origin of the perforator vessels, a careful dissection was carried out along the perforators to the skin paddle, while saving all the branches to the VL muscle flap. Various sizes of the VL muscle were harvested with the ALT flap, depending on the ideal reconstruction of various defects. The skin and muscular components of the flap—each provided by a separate branch—can be easily placed into the defect thanks to the mobility of the pedicle.

When harvesting the muscle flap, a harmonic scalpel (Ethicon Endo-Surgery, Cincinnati, OH, USA) was used to minimize bleeding and shorten the operation time. En block elevation of the ALT skin flap and VL muscle flap was performed. The descending branch of the lateral circumflex femoral vessel was dissected further in a proximal direction. The harvested chimeric flap (Figure 1A,B), skin paddle, and muscle segment were placed side by side in parallel, and the abutting margin was secured in place with Vicryl #3-0 sutures to prevent separation. Next, the conjoined chimeric flap was transferred to the defect site and the flap was temporarily fixed for stable vascular anastomosis. After vascular anastomosis, we carefully checked that there was no pulling or twisting of the main pedicle or the pedicle to each segment. The margin of the flap was checked for its viability by observing it for fresh bleeding. A split thickness skin graft was performed to cover the VL muscle segment. The flap was clinically monitored using the refilling test and clinical evaluation of the skin paddle flap colour and temperature. Between the fourth and fifth postoperative day, the split thickness skin graft was opened and checked to confirm whether the graft was successful. From week 1 after surgery, the patients were mobile.

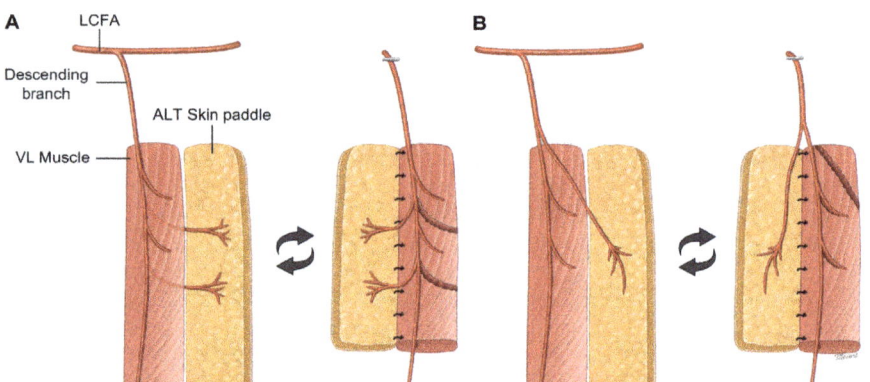

Figure 1. Schematic illustration of an anterolateral thigh (ALT)/vastus lateralis (VL) chimeric flap. (**A**) The musculocutaneous perforator to ALT flap is dissected at the intramuscular level between the VL muscles. The VL muscle flap is elevated on the muscular branch of the same vessel. (**B**) The ALT flap is harvested after complete dissection of the perforator, which travels briefly through the muscle, proximal to the VL muscle. Separate pedicles are directed to the VL muscle flap.

3. Results

Ten patients were included in the present study; their characteristics are summarized in Table 1. Their ages ranged from 16 to 63 years, with an average of 47.7 years. Five participants were male and five were female. The aetiology was trauma ($n = 3$), tumour ($n = 6$), and infection ($n = 1$); the locations included the lower leg ($n = 3$), trunk ($n = 5$), and knee joint ($n = 2$).

The flap remained 100% viable in all patients. All defects were fully covered by the ALT/VL chimeric flap, and donor sites were closed by a primary closure in all patients. Two patients underwent radiotherapy after surgery. Hospital discharge occurred between 16 and 21 days after surgery with a mean hospitalization time of 18 days. All patients were followed up at 6 months and 1 year. The average width of the ALT flaps harvested from the ten patients was 8.6 cm (6–10 cm). The average width of the VL flaps harvested from the ten patients was 9.0 cm (7–10 cm). The average pedicle length was 7.1 cm (5–10 cm). In one case, a vein graft was necessary to elongate the pedicle length.

No major complications were encountered. One case had a minor graft site complication that resulted in unstable hypertrophic scarring on the split-thickness skin of the VL muscle area. One patient experienced flap bulkiness, which improved after subsequent liposuction. The patients did not experience any difficulty with walking or running. The results were satisfactory at the last follow-up.

Table 1. Demographic information of patients who underwent ALT & VL chimeric flap.

Patient No.	Gender	Age	Diagnosis	Location	ALT Size (cm)	VL Size (cm)	Total Flap Size (cm)	Pedicle Length (cm)
1	M	63	Sarcoma	Trunk	16 × 6	15 × 10	27 × 20	5
2	F	63	SCC	Knee joint	14 × 8	18 × 10	26 × 25	5
3	F	16	Infection	Lower leg	14 × 8	10 × 8	22 × 18	7
4	M	58	SCC	Lower leg	15 × 10	11 × 8	25 × 18	9
5	F	38	Trauma	Trunk	13 × 9	10 × 9	23 × 18	6
6	M	28	Scar contracture	Knee joint	15 × 10	11 × 10	20 × 15	8
7	F	44	Trauma	Lower leg	15 × 10	10 × 9	25 × 10	6
8	M	32	DFSP	trunk	11 × 7	9 × 7	18 × 14	8
9	F	63	Fibrosarcoma	Trunk	13 × 10	10 × 9	23 × 17	10
10	M	72	Osteosarcoma	Trunk	12 × 8	13 × 10	25 × 16	7
Average		47.7						7.1

ALT, anterolateral thigh; VL, vastus lateralis; SCC, squamous cell carcinoma; DFSP, dermatofibromasarcoma protuberans.

3.1. Case Reports

3.1.1. Case 1

A 63-year-old male patient presented with a recurrent known malignant peripheral nerve sheath tumour infiltrating the posterior trunk region. Under general anaesthesia and in the prone position, the lesion was resected with a 3 cm margin. The size of the resultant defect was 16.0 × 15.0 cm (Figure 2A) with rib exposure. For defect reconstruction, the patient was placed in the supine position and the ALT/VL chimeric flap was elevated with skin and muscular components of 6.0 × 16.0 and 10.0 × 15.0 cm, respectively (Figure 2B). The autologous vein graft was harvested to elongate the pedicle length from the great saphenous vein. Defects were reconstructed as described previously, and the patient healed uneventfully (Figure 2C,D).

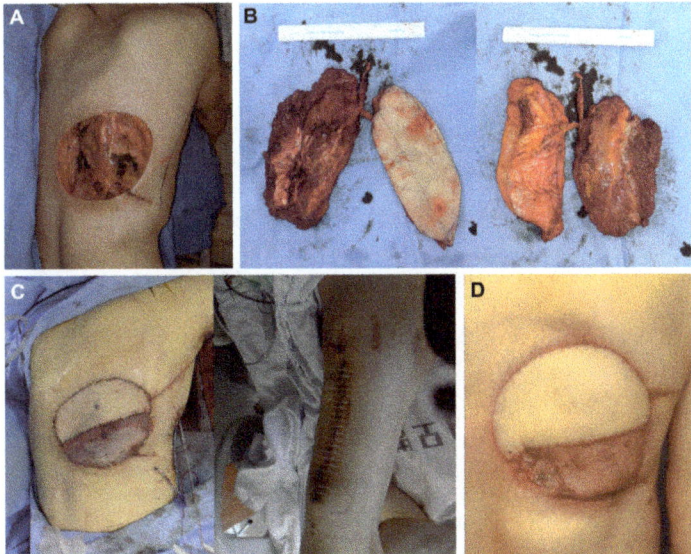

Figure 2. (Case 1). (**A**) Large defect size (16 × 15 cm) on the posterior trunk lesion after wide excision. (**B**) Harvested anterolateral thigh (ALT)/vastus lateralis (VL) chimeric flap. (**C**) Flap inset and immediate postoperative photo of the donor site. (**D**) Clinical photo at 4 months post-operation.

3.1.2. Case 2

A 63-year-old female presented with a Marjolin's ulcer originating from the right popliteal area (Figure 3A). A wide excision was performed, leaving an extensive defect size of 15.0 × 20.0 cm (Figure 3B). An ALT/VL chimeric flap was harvested from the left thigh with skin and muscular components of 7.0 × 20.0 and 8.0 × 18.0 cm, respectively (Figure 3C). The skin paddles and muscular components for the flaps were placed side by side to cover the skin surface of the soft-tissue defect of the right knee. The donor sites were closed directly. After anastomosis, an intraoperative Indocyanine Green Angiography (ICG) study showed that the flap circulation was intact (Figure 3D). All flaps survived completely. The recipient site presented a satisfactory contour (Figure 3E,F). The patient was able to ambulate fully with no apparent functional deficits related to the donor site at their last follow-up visit 12 months after the operation.

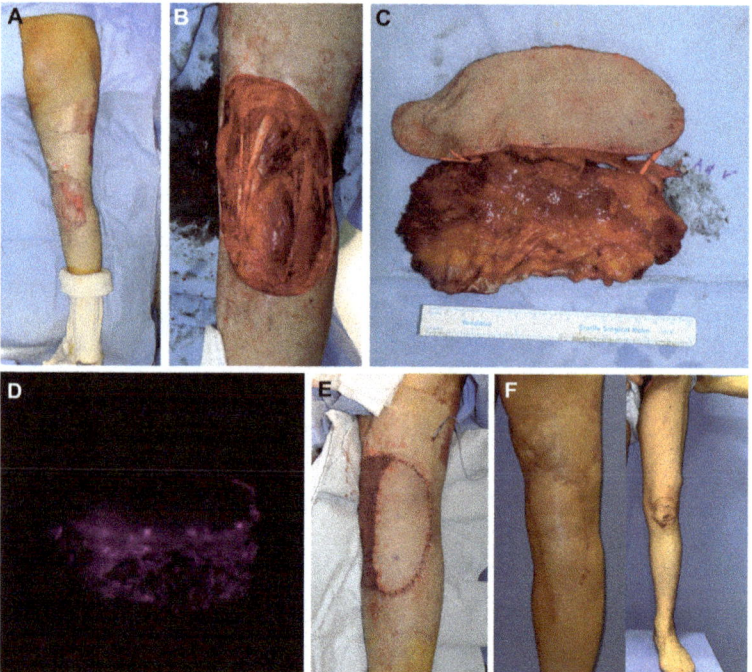

Figure 3. (Case 2). (**A**) Preoperative clinical photo before wide excision. (**B**) Extensive defect size (15 × 20 cm) on the right popliteal area. (**C**) Harvested anterolateral thigh (ALT)/vastus lateralis (VL) chimeric flap. (**D**) The Indocyanine Green Angiography (ICG) fluoroscopy of the harvested flap shows stable illumination of both the ALT skin flap and VL muscle flap. (**E**) Postoperative clinical photo immediately after ALT/VL flap coverage. (**F**) Clinical photo at 12 months post-operation. The flap was well incorporated, and the donor site healed well.

3.1.3. Case 3

A 17-year-old female patient suffered from leukaemia that caused skin and soft tissue necrosis in the right lower leg (Figure 4A). After radical debridement, the resultant defect was 37.0 × 19.0 cm with tibial exposure (Figure 4B). An ALT/VL chimeric flap was microsurgically harvested to reconstruct the extensive defect in one stage. The skin paddle of the flap and the muscle component dimensions were 37.0 × 8.0 cm and 20.0 × 8.0 cm, respectively (Figure 4C). The skin paddle of the flaps and muscle components were placed side by side to cover the defect. Above the muscle component, a split-thickness skin graft was performed (Figure 4D). The postoperative course was uneventful. The recipient site showed a satisfactory contour and mild bulkiness of the flap site led to considerations for possible fat injection for contour correction in the future (Figure 4E).

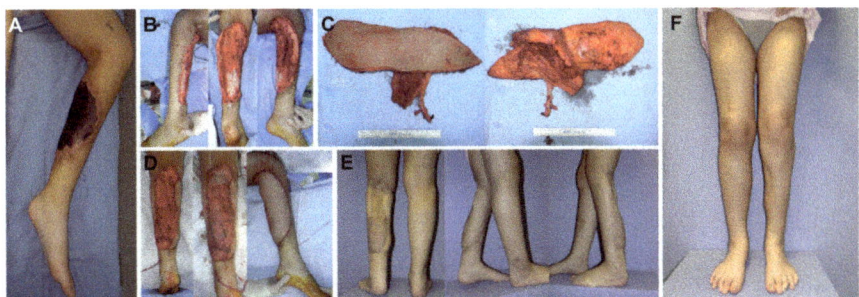

Figure 4. (Case 3). (**A**) Skin and soft tissue necrosis involving the right lower leg. (**B**) Large defect size (37 × 19 cm) after radical debridement. (**C**) Harvested anterolateral (ALT)/vastus lateralis (VL) chimeric flap. (**D**) Immediate postoperative clinical photo. (**E,F**) Postoperative clinical photo at 12 months post-operation.

4. Discussion

The present study analysed a series of ten cases of reconstruction for complex large defects using the ALT/VL chimeric flap in one stage. We demonstrated that this is a safe and reliable alternative option for the reconstruction of large defects in various cases.

Traditionally, various free flaps, such as the LD, TRAM, and ALT, have been used for the reconstruction of extensive large defects [9,22–26]. Among these flaps, the ALT free flap is well known and has been used as a standard flap due to its advantages, such as the easy anatomical approach to pedicles and relatively easy harvesting [6,7,23]. However, when the defect is very large, the ALT flap alone may not be able to cover the defect.

In general, the ALT/VL chimeric flap cannot be selected as the first choice for wide defect coverage. However, it may be selected as an alternative option in the following cases. First, this method may be used when TRAM or LD flaps are contraindicated or when patients refuse a donor-site scar in the abdomen or trunk area. Second, this method may be used in cases where an ALT flap alone is planned initially, but the defect area is larger than expected and the ALT flap alone is inadequate to cover the defect. Harvesting the wider skin flap is possible in the ALT, but in this case, an additional microanastomosis process of turbocharging or supercharging must be performed to incorporate anteromedial thigh (AMT) perforators into the flap. Third, this method may be used in cases where the defect area is less sensitive than the donor site of thigh lesions, such as trunk lesions.

A chimeric perforator flap consisting of independent tissue flaps, such as skin flaps and muscle flaps with their own independent vascular supply linked to a common vascular source, has many advantages in covering extensive tissue defects [6,27–32].

The ALT flap is a perforator and intermittent septocutaneous flap provided by the lateral cutaneous perforator of the descending branch of the LCFA, which is a branch of the deep femoral artery [1,4,17]. The VL muscle is a type I muscle predominantly supplied by the same descending branch of the ALT flap, although it can also be fed by the transverse branches of the LCFA [21,22,33]. This vascular anatomy enables the ALT and VL muscle flaps to be elevated as a chimeric flap.

The advantages of harvesting the ALT/VL chimeric flaps to reconstruct extensive tissue defects are as follows. First, the chimeric flap provides a large amount of soft tissue and multiple flap components that an individual flap cannot provide; therefore, extensive defects can be covered using the chimeric flap in one stage [6,31,33]. Second, donor site primary closure is possible, which yields better aesthetic results and minimizes donor site morbidity. Third, the ALT/VL chimeric flap can be elevated simultaneously without the need for patient repositioning. Moreover, only one pair of recipient vessels is required to supply the entire chimeric flap. When we compare the ALT/VL chimeric flap with the ALT turbocharged flap with an AMT perforator [23], no additional microsurgical anastomosis is necessary; therefore, this technique consumes less time, and a more straightforward flap harvesting is possible.

Although the ALT/VL chimeric flap has many benefits in the reconstruction of extensive tissue defects, there are several disadvantages to this method. First, the use of the ALT/VL chimeric flap requires a longer learning curve and technical difficulty is high. Second, this technique requires the coverage of a skin graft on top of the VL muscle flap, which may cause contour deformity and create an aesthetically unfavourable outcome. Third, the ALT flap presents variable anatomy [19,20,23], where muscular dissection is necessary in most cases, increasing the operation time. In addition, there may be no perforator vessels arising from the descending branch of the lateral circumflex to the skin flap. However, even in these cases, it is possible to harvest a chimeric flap based not on perforators but on the entire descending branch of the LCFA with the segment of the VL muscle as needed.

In this study, we focused on assessing the outcomes of the chimeric flap technique for the reconstruction of large soft tissue defects. However, it is important to note that we did not directly compare these outcomes with those of conventional large skin flaps of the ALT under identical conditions. This represents a significant limitation of our study, as a direct comparative analysis would have provided valuable insights into the relative advantages and disadvantages of these two surgical approaches. Further studies with a large patient group and long-term follow-up are needed to assess the effectiveness of this technique.

5. Conclusions

The novel ALT/VL chimeric flap is a safe, effective, and well-tolerated method with acceptable donor site morbidity. This makes the ALT/VL chimeric flap a useful alternative for the reconstruction of wide extensive defects in various cases. In our study, no major complications were observed, with encouraging functional and aesthetic outcomes.

Author Contributions: Conceptualization, Y.J.L. and S.-H.M.; methodology, J.K. and S.-H.M.; software, C.R.L. and J.K.; validation, Y.J.L., Y.J.J. and S.-H.M.; formal analysis, J.H.K. and S.-H.M.; investigation, J.H.K. and D.Y.O.; resources, S.-H.M.; data curation, C.R.L.; writing—original draft preparation, Y.J.L.; writing—review and editing, S.-H.M.; visualization, J.K.; supervision, S.-H.M.; project administration, S.-H.M.; funding acquisition, S.-H.M. All authors have read and agreed to the published version of the manuscript.

Funding: This work was supported by the Korea Medical Device Development Fund grant funded by the Korea government (the Ministry of Science and ICT, Information and Communication Technology, the Ministry of Health & Welfare, the Ministry of Food and Drug Safety) (Project Number: 202012E02).

Institutional Review Board Statement: The study was conducted under local ethical committee approval, Committee of the Catholic University of Korea (KC23RISI0779) and conducted in accordance with ethical standards of the Declaration of Helsinki.

Informed Consent Statement: Signing informed consent was not required based on the conducted analysis, due to the retrospective nature of the study, the fully anonymized set of clinical data, and in accordance with the Ethics Committee's decision.

Data Availability Statement: The data can be obtained by scientists who conduct work independently from the industry, on request. The data are not stored on publicly available servers.

Conflicts of Interest: The authors declare no conflict of interest.

References

1. Kuo, Y.R.; Jeng, S.F.; Kuo, M.H.; Huang, M.N.; Liu, Y.T.; Chiang, Y.C.; Yeh, M.C.; Wei, F.C. Free anterolateral thigh flap for extremity reconstruction: Clinical experience and functional assessment of donor site. *Plast. Reconstr. Surg.* **2001**, *107*, 1766–1771. [CrossRef] [PubMed]
2. Wei, F.C.; Jain, V.; Celik, N.; Chen, H.C.; Chuang, D.C.; Lin, C.H. Have we found an ideal soft-tissue flap? An experience with 672 anterolateral thigh flaps. *Plast. Reconstr. Surg.* **2002**, *109*, 2219–2226; discussion 2227–2230. [CrossRef] [PubMed]

3. Kimata, Y.; Uchiyama, K.; Ebihara, S.; Sakuraba, M.; Iida, H.; Nakatsuka, T.; Harii, K. Anterolateral thigh flap donor—Site complication and mortality. *Plast. Reconstr. Surg.* **2000**, *106*, 584–589. [CrossRef]
4. Lee, J.H.; Chung, D.W.; Han, C.S. Outcomes of anterolateral thigh-free flaps and conversion from external to internal fixation with bone grafting in gustilo type IIIB open tibial fractures. *Microsurgery* **2012**, *32*, 431–437. [CrossRef]
5. Kwee, M.M.; Rozen, W.M.; Ting, J.W.; Mirkazemi, M.; Leong, J.; Baillieu, C. Total scalp reconstruction with bilateral anterolateral thigh flaps. *Microsurgery* **2012**, *32*, 393–396. [CrossRef]
6. Ng, S.W.; Fong, H.C.; Tan, B.K. Two sequential free flaps for coverage of a total knee implant. *Arch. Plast. Surg.* **2018**, *45*, 280–283. [CrossRef] [PubMed]
7. Jo, G.Y.; Ki, S.H. Analysis of the chest wall reconstruction methods after malignant tumor resection. *Arch. Plast. Surg.* **2023**, *50*, 10–16. [CrossRef] [PubMed]
8. Kato, S.; Sakuma, H.; Fujii, T.; Tanaka, I.; Matsui, J. Reconstruction of extensive diaphragmatic defects using the rectus abdominis muscle and fascial flap. *Arch. Plast. Surg.* **2023**, *50*, 166–170. [CrossRef]
9. Gaster, R.S.; Bhatt, K.A.; Shelton, A.A.; Lee, G.K. Free transverse rectus abdominis myocutaneous flap reconstruction of a massive lumbosacral defect using superior gluteal artery perforator vessels. *Microsurgery* **2012**, *32*, 388–392. [CrossRef]
10. Lee, Y.J.; Baek, S.E.; Lee, J.; Oh, D.Y.; Rhie, J.W.; Moon, S.H. Perforating vessel as an alternative option of a recipient selection for posterior trunk-free flap reconstruction. *Microsurgery* **2018**, *38*, 763–771. [CrossRef]
11. Abraham, J.T.; Saint-Cyr, M. Keystone and pedicle perforator flaps in reconstructive surgery: New modifications and applications. *Clin. Plast. Surg.* **2017**, *44*, 385–402. [CrossRef] [PubMed]
12. Jo, G.Y.; Yoon, J.M.; Ki, S.H. Reconstruction of a large chest wall defect using bilateral pectoralis major myocutaneous flaps and V-Y rotation advancement flaps: A case report. *Arch. Plast. Surg.* **2022**, *49*, 39–42. [CrossRef] [PubMed]
13. Gierek, M.; Klama-Baryla, A.; Labus, W.; Bergler-Czop, B.; Pietrauszka, K.; Niemiec, P. Platelet-Rich Plasma and Acellular Dermal Matrix in the Surgical Treatment of Hidradenitis Suppurativa: A Comparative Restrospective Study. *J. Clin. Med.* **2023**, *14*, 2112. [CrossRef] [PubMed]
14. Gierek, M.; Labus, W.; Kitala, D.; Lorek, A.; Ochala-Gierek, G.; Zagorska, K.; Waniczek, D.; Szyluk, K.; Niemiec, P. Human Acellular Dermal Matrix in Reconstructive Surgery—A Review. *Biomedicines* **2022**, *10*, 2870. [CrossRef]
15. Gierek, M.; Labus, W.; Slabon, A.; Ziokowska, K.; Ochala-Gierek, G.; Kitala, D.; Szyluk, K.; Niemiec, P. Co-Graft of Acellular Dermal Matrix and Split Thickness Skin Graft-A New Reconstructive Surgical Method in the Treatment of Hidradenitis Suppurativa. *Bioengineering* **2022**, *9*, 389. [CrossRef]
16. Heo, C.Y.; Kang, B.; Jeong, J.H.; Kim, K.; Myung, Y. Acellular dermal matrix and bone cement sandwich technique for chest wall reconstruction. *Arch. Plast. Surg.* **2022**, *49*, 25–28. [CrossRef]
17. Koshima, I.; Hosoda, M.; Moriguchi, T.; Hamanaka, T.; Kawata, S.; Hata, T. A combined anterolateral thigh flap, anteromedial thigh flap, and vascularized iliac bone graft for a full-thickness defect of the mental region. *Ann. Plast. Surg.* **1993**, *31*, 175–180. [CrossRef]
18. Koshima, I.; Yamamoto, H.; Hosoda, M.; Moriguchi, T.; Orita, Y.; Nagayama, H. Free combined composite flaps using the lateral circumflex femoral system for repair of massive defects of the head and neck regions: An introduction to the chimeric flap principle. *Plast. Reconstr. Surg.* **1993**, *92*, 411–420. [CrossRef]
19. Kimata, Y.; Uchiyama, K.; Ebihara, S.; Yoshizumi, T.; Asai, M.; Saikawa, M.; Hayashi, R.; Jitsuiki, Y.; Majima, K.; Ohyama, W.; et al. Versatility of the free anterolateral thigh flap for reconstruction of head and neck defects. *Arch. Otolaryngol. Head. Neck Surg.* **1997**, *123*, 1325–1331. [CrossRef]
20. Graboyes, E.M.; Hornig, J.D. Evolution of the anterolateral thigh free flap. *Curr. Opin. Otolaryngol. Head. Neck Surg.* **2017**, *25*, 416–421. [CrossRef]
21. Yang, R.; Wu, X.; Kumar, P.A.; Xiong, Y.; Jiang, C.; Jian, X.; Guo, F. Application of chimerical ALT perforator flap with vastus lateralis muscle mass for the reconstruction of oral and submandibular defects after radical resection of tongue carcinoma: A retrospective cohort study. *BMC Oral Health* **2020**, *20*, 94. [CrossRef]
22. Kim, S.W.; Kim, K.N.; Hong, J.P.; Park, S.W.; Park, C.R.; Yoon, C.S. Use of the chimeric anterolateral thigh free flap in lower extremity reconstruction. *Microsurgery* **2015**, *35*, 634–639. [CrossRef]
23. Wong, C.H.; Wei, F.C. Anterolateral thigh flap. *Head Neck* **2010**, *32*, 529–540. [CrossRef] [PubMed]
24. Lee, Y.J.; Lee, Y.J.; Oh, D.Y.; Jun, Y.J.; Rhie, J.W.; Moon, S.H. Reconstruction of wide soft tissue defects with extended anterolateral thigh perforator flap turbocharged technique with anteromedial thigh perforator. *Microsurgery* **2020**, *40*, 440–446. [CrossRef] [PubMed]
25. Lee, K.T.; Wiraatmadja, E.S.; Mun, G.H. Free latissimus dorsi muscle-chimeric thoracodorsal artery perforator flaps for reconstruction of complicated defects: Does muscle still have a place in the domain of perforator flaps? *Ann. Plast. Surg.* **2015**, *74*, 565–572. [CrossRef] [PubMed]
26. Hallock, G.G. The role of free flaps for salvage of the exposed total ankle arthroplasty. *Microsurgery* **2017**, *37*, 34–37. [CrossRef]
27. Yamamoto, T.; Yamamoto, N.; Ishiura, R. Free double-paddle superficial circumflex iliac perforator flap transfer for partial maxillectomy reconstruction: A case report. *Microsurgery* **2022**, *42*, 84–88. [CrossRef] [PubMed]
28. Low, O.-W.; Loh, T.; Lee, H.; Yap, Y.; Lim, J.; Lim, T.; Nallathamby, V. The superior lateral genicular artery flap for reconstruction of knee and proximal leg defect. *Arch. Plast. Surg.* **2022**, *49*, 108–114. [CrossRef]

29. Cannady, S.B.; Mady, L.J.; Brody, R.M.; Shimunov, D.; Newman, J.G.; Chalian, A.C.; Rajasekaran, K.A.; Sheth, N.P.; Shanti, R.M. Anterolateral thigh osteomyocutaneous flap in head and neck: Lessons learned. *Microsurgery* **2022**, *42*, 117–124. [CrossRef]
30. Scaglioni, M.F.; Meroni, M.; Knobe, M.; Fritsche, E. Versatility of perforator flaps for lower extremity defect coverage: Technical highlights and single center experience with 87 consecutive cases. *Microsurgery* **2022**, *42*, 548–556. [CrossRef]
31. Hallock, G.G. Further clarification of the nomenclature for compound flaps. *Plast. Reconstr. Surg.* **2006**, *117*, 151e–160e. [CrossRef] [PubMed]
32. Hallock, G.G. The complete nomenclature for combined perforator flaps. *Plast. Reconstr. Surg.* **2011**, *127*, 1720–1729. [CrossRef] [PubMed]
33. Simsek, T.; Engin, M.S.; Yildirim, K.; Kodalak, E.A.; Demir, A. Reconstruction of extensive orbital exenteration defects using an anterolateral thigh/vastus lateralis chimeric flap. *J. Craniofac. Surg.* **2017**, *28*, 638–642. [CrossRef] [PubMed]

Disclaimer/Publisher's Note: The statements, opinions and data contained in all publications are solely those of the individual author(s) and contributor(s) and not of MDPI and/or the editor(s). MDPI and/or the editor(s) disclaim responsibility for any injury to people or property resulting from any ideas, methods, instructions or products referred to in the content.

Article
Reliability of Long Vein Grafts for Reconstruction of Massive Wounds

Brian Chuong [1,*], Kristopher Katira [2,*], Taylor Ramsay [3], John LoGiudice [4,*] and Antony Martin [2]

1. College of Science Main Campus, University of Utah, Salt Lake City, UT 84112, USA
2. Intermountain Healthcare, Salt Lake City, UT 84107, USA
3. Salt Lake Community College, Main Campus, Salt Lake City, UT 84123, USA
4. Department of Plastic and Reconstructive Surgery, Medical College of Wisconsin, Milwaukee, WI 53226, USA
* Correspondence: brian116c@gmail.com (B.C.); kmk3361@gmail.com (K.K.); jlogiudice@mcw.edu (J.L.)

Abstract: When handling large wounds, zone of injury is a key concept in reconstructive microsurgery, as it pertains to the selection of recipient vessels. Historically, surgeons have avoided placing microvascular anastomosis within widely traumatized, inflamed, or radiated fields. The harvest of vein grafts facilitates reconstruction in complex cases by extending arterial and/or venous pedicle length. To illustrate the utility and fidelity of these techniques, this paper reviews the indications and outcomes for vein grafting in ten consecutive patients at a single tertiary referral center hospital. The case series presented is unique in three aspects. First, there are two cases of successful coaptation of the flap artery to the side of the arterial limb of an arteriovenous loop. Second, there is a large proportion of cases where vein grafts were used to elongate the venous pedicle. In these 10 cases, the mean vein graft length was 37 cm. We observed zero flap failures and zero amputations. Although limited in sample size, these case data support the efficacy and reliability of long segment vein grafting in complex cases in referral centers.

Keywords: microsurgery; plastic surgery; free flap reconstruction; AV loops; end-to-side anastomoses

1. Introduction

Microsurgery is the technical means through which free tissue transfer is accomplished. In large cancer and trauma referral centers, free tissue transfer involves using skin, muscle, and/or bone to restore massive soft tissue defects in the head and neck, trunk, and extremities. Naturally, executing a free flap requires meticulous planning, including careful flap and recipient vessel selection [1]. "Zone of injury" is a critical concept in this context, as heavily scarred, traumatized, or poorly perfused vessels do not nourish or drain a free flap, potentially leading to the dreaded complication of flap failure. In this regard, vein grafting is an important yet often under-recognized tool for successfully reconstructing even the most complex and heavily damaged wounds [2].

The following manuscript describes a case series of ten consecutive patients in a single tertiary referral center in which free tissue transfer was used to restore traumatic or oncologic defects. Descriptive details of the procedures, employed techniques, length of vein grafts used, and outcomes are provided as evidence of the efficacy, reliability, and reproducibility of large segment vein grafting in even the most intricate reconstructive cases. To bolster the significance of these findings, the outcomes from our case series are juxtaposed against the existing literature on long vein graft free flap tissue transfers [3–7]. In these referenced articles, patients underwent various forms of free tissue transfer involving vein grafting, with discussions on indications, complications, and success rates. This comparative analysis underscores the high levels of success in each of the cases presented, providing valuable insight and reinforcement into the utility of vein grafting as a vital tool in the arsenal of microsurgeons.

2. Methods

Ten consecutive patient charts at a single institution (Intermountain Medical Center) over a two-year period were studied to elucidate details about the nature of the problems requiring reconstruction, the technical details of the operation, the size of the wounds, and the length of the vein grafts used. Complications such as hematoma, flap loss, microvascular thrombosis, re-operation, and time to soft tissue healing were recorded and tabulated. Institutional review board approval was obtained for the recording and publication of these data (ID: 1052396). All patient photos were de-identified to the fullest extent possible. Written consent for photograph release and for publication of these data were obtained.

Vein grafts were used when flaps could not be inset using standard pedicle lengths, especially in cases involving heavily traumatized, scarred, or radiated fields. Consent was obtained from patients pre-operatively. Sonographic vein mapping was performed in one case using vascular lab services. Perioperative chemoprophylaxis was routinely administered. Non-constrictive and well-padded splinting was employed in cases involving extremities to avoid motion when long vein grafts spanned joint soft tissues. Vein grafts used were typically inset under wide subcutaneous tunnels to allow coaptation to recipient vessels. Arteriovenous (AV) loops were allowed flowing for at least 30 min before division, enabling the correction of vasospasm prior to flap coaptation.

3. Results

Figures 1–4 depict cases in which long vein grafts were employed for various defects. The indications and techniques in this consecutive series of 10 patients are summarized in Table 1. The mean vein graft length was 37 cm. The most common vein graft donor site length was the thigh's greater saphenous vein (9/10 cases). The most common flap used was the anterolateral thigh flap (ALT, N = 4), followed by latissimus (N = 2), vastus lateralis (N = 2), followed by gracilis (N = 1) and radial forearm (N = 1). Flap viability was 100% with a minimum follow-up of 3 months and a maximum follow-up of 18 months. Amputation was avoided in 100% of patients during this time. Nine cases were related to acute or subacute traumatic defects (within the same hospitalization as the index traumatic injury), and one case was related to radiation injury. One trauma-related case was several years removed from the injury.

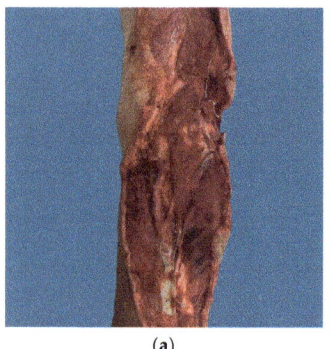
(a)

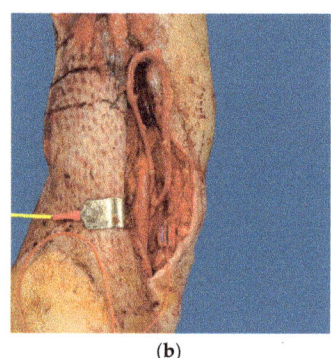
(b)

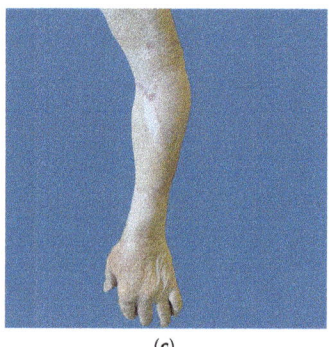
(c)

Figure 1. Patient B in Tables 1 and 2. Free tissue transfer was performed for definitive wound coverage after extensive and prolonged degloving injury, allowing for future reconstructions of PIN palsy. A pedicled latissimus flap was used to cover a Gustilo Grade IIIa condylar fracture prior to attempting free tissue transfer, allowing for skin paddle placement over an antibiotic spacer. Dermal matrix was used to temporize the distal wound bed before free tissue transfer. (**a**) Defect; (**b**) Arteriovenous (AV) Loop creation; (**c**) 1 year follow-up.

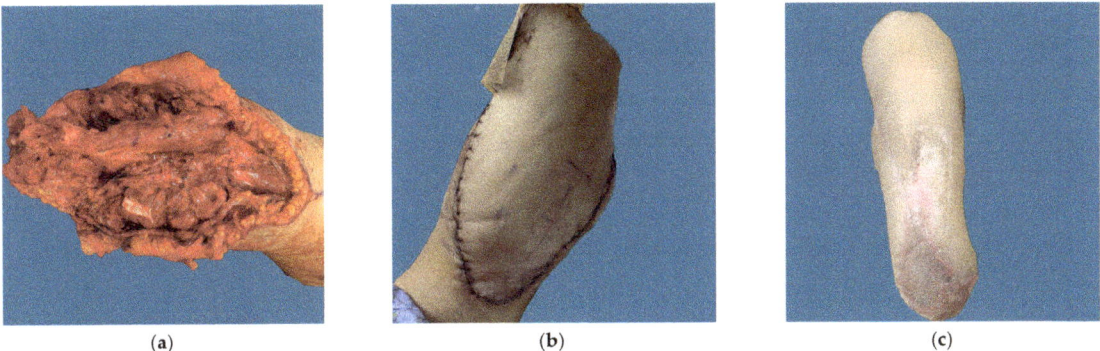

Figure 2. Patient D in Tables 1 and 2. Industrial accident resulting in trans-radial amputation. A traditional AV loop was created to allow for elbow preservation and prosthetic fitting. (**a**) Defect with AV loop; (**b**) Immediate post op result after ALT flap; (**c**) Healed flap/skin graft at 6 months.

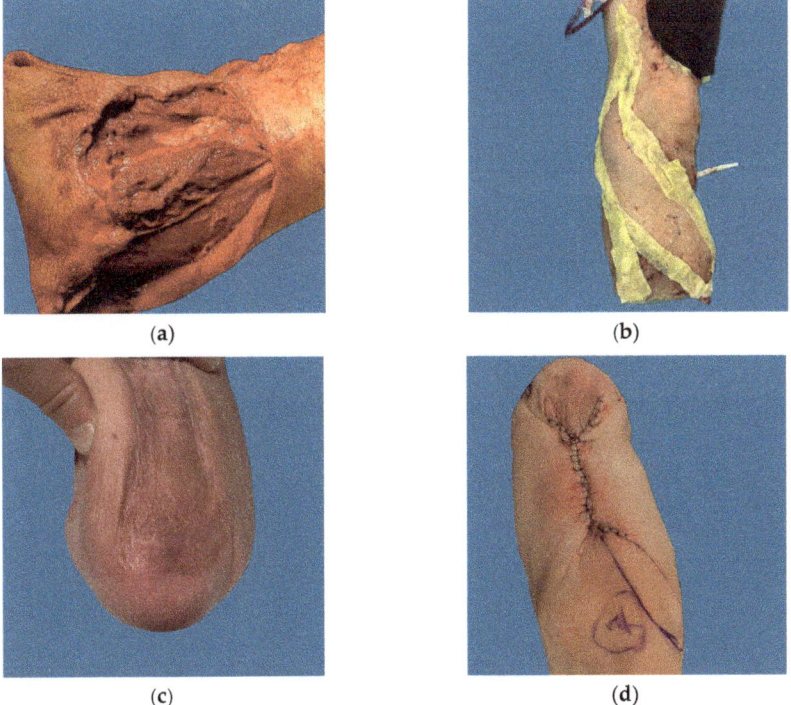

Figure 3. Patient A in Tables 1 and 2. Pedestrian versus automobile accident resulting in traumatic amputation. (**a**) After internal fixation and antibiotic spacer; (**b**) Myocutaneous free tissue transfer was performed to preserve the below-knee amputation stump; (**c**,**d**) Flap elevation and advancement after Masquelet bone grafting.

Table 1. Indications and Technique for Vein Graft Anastomosis.

Patient	Etiology	Indication	Location (Size, cm)	Flap	Vein Graft (cm)	Recipient Artery/Vein	Technique (Figure 5)
A	Pedestrian vs. MVC	IIIB Open Fracture	Anterior BKA Stump	MC Vastus Lateralis	GSV (25) Leg and Thigh	Medial Genicular a./GSV	Type 2
B	MVA Degloving	IIIA Open Fracture, PIN Palsy	Elbow Forearm, Arm	ALT	GSV (35)	Brachial a./Brachial V.	Type 3
C	MVA Degloving	IIIB Open Fracture	Circumferential Forearm	Latissimus	GSV (44)	Radial a./Brachial V.	Type 1
D	Industrial Machine	IIIC Fracture, Multiple Nerves Injured	Forearm	ALT	GSV (50)	Proximal Ulnar a./Brachial V.	Type 3
E	Sarcoma	Radiation	Tibia, Knee	Vastus Lateralis	GSV (70) Leg and Thigh	LCF a. and TFL Branch a./GSV	Type 4 for Artery Type 1 for Vein
F	Industrial Machine	Soft Tissue Degloving, Ulnar Nerve and Flexor Tendon Injuries	Wrist, Forearm	ALT	GSV (33)	Ulnar a./Brachial V.	ES a. Type 1 Vein
G	Infection	Exposed Tendon, Median Nerve	Wrist	ALT	LFC vc (25)	Radial a./Brachial V.	EE a. Type 1 Vein
H	Blast	Degloved Thumb	Hand	Gracilis	GSV (30)	Radial a./Radial V.C.	ES a. Type 1 Vein
I	Blast	Distal Third Extremity Wound, Remote Injury	Ankle	Radial Forearm	GSV (30)	Posterior Tibial a. Superficial Vein	EE a. Type 1 Vein

Index of Table 1: MVC—Motor Vehicle Collision. LFC—Lateral Femoral Circumflex. TFL—Tensor Fascia Lata. VC—Vena Comitans. ES—End to Side. EE—End to End. AV—Arteriovenous. PIN—Posterior Interosseous Nerve. BKA—Below the Knee Amputation. MC—Musculocutaneous. ALT—Anterolateral Thigh Flap. GSV—Greater Saphenous Vein.

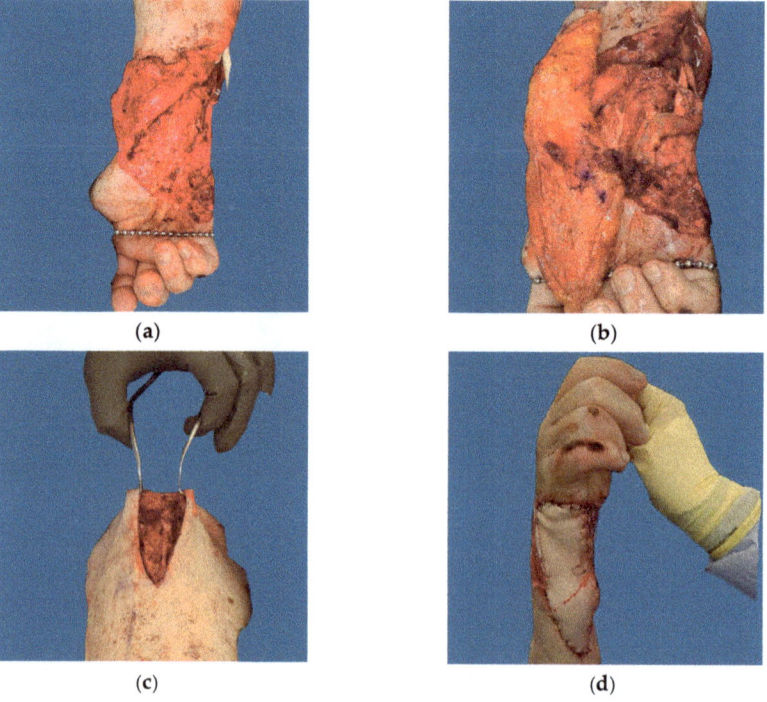

Figure 4. Patient F in Tables 1 and 2. Extensive crush mechanism resulting in exposure of the ulnar nerve with flexor tendon injury. A long vein graft was used to bridge the flap vein to more proximal veins, providing outflow to large competent vessels outside of the zone of injury; (**a**) Defect; (**b**,**c**) Vein graft used to extend venous pedicle from flap to uninjured proximal antebrachial vein; (**d**) Final inset.

Table 2. Complications and Outcome Vein Graft.

Patient	Takeback for Anastomosis Revision	Other Takeback	Thromboembolism (DVT/PE)	Soft Tissue Healed?	Post-Operative Amputation?	Follow-Up (Months)
A	Yes; Washout hematoma, thrombectomy, vein revision, washout and closure of flap donor site	Yes; Secondary Orthopedic Procedures	No	Yes	No	18
B	No	Yes; Skin Grafting of Wound, Excision of Neuroma	No	Yes	No	12
C	No	Yes; Donor Site Infection	No	Yes	No	12
D	No	No	No	Yes	No	6
E	Yes; washout hematoma, thrombectomy, vein revision	No	No	Yes	No	3
F	No	No	No	Yes	No	12
G	No	No	No	Yes	No	9
H	No	No	No	Yes	No	12
I	No	No	No	Yes	No	6

Table 1 summarizes the indications, etiologies, and technical aspects of wound coverage in this series. Two surgical teams were used to execute these cases. A variety of vein graft techniques were employed, including three cases of traditional arteriovenous (AV) loop, two of which required end-to-side anastomosis of the flap vessel along the arterial limb of the vein graft. Two AV loop cases were connected to free flaps in a single stage, while the remaining case was performed in two stages to allow for scheduling of a definitive free flap. In the two-stage arteriovenous (AV) flap, the AV loops was left in place under skin flaps and then divided in a separate procedure. The two-stage technique in this case was applied for purely logistical reasons.

Table 2 summarizes complications and outcomes related to these flap transfers. Unplanned takeback occurred in two patients due to venous anastomotic revision. In Patient A, two takebacks were required for drainage of flap site hematoma on Postoperative day (POD) 1 and venous revision on POD 2. Additionally, two procedures were performed for donor site wound closure and dermal regeneration template grafting in the same hospitalization. Patient E also required takeback for hematoma and revision of the venous anastomosis on POD 1. Patient C had one unplanned takeback following discharge to wash out a donor site seroma. Patient A also underwent skin grafting of a dermal regeneration template and two secondary orthopedic procedures after hospital discharge. There were no cases of major venous thromboembolism, flap loss, or revision amputation during the follow-up periods. The minimum follow-up was three months for one patient, while the rest of the patients had a follow-up duration of six months or more.

Multiple types of AV looping techniques exist. Type 1 construct consisted of a flap vein sewn or coupled end to end to a vein graft, and the downstream limb of the vein graft was then sewn or coupled end to end to the recipient vein. There was a total of seven Type 1 vein grafts in seven patients. All seven cases were for efferent connections.

Type 2 and Type 3 constructs comprised the arteriovenous loop vein graft group. Type 2 involved creation of a traditional AV loop, in which an end-to-end connection was formed between the vein graft and the recipient artery and vein. This loop was then divided in the same surgery (one-stage AV loop) or in a separate procedure (two-stage), creating afferent and efferent vein segments which were then connected end to end to flap vessels. Type 3 involved a size-mismatched AV loop. In this type, a standard AV loop was created as in Type 2. Unlike Type 2, however, the flap artery was sewn end to side, rather than end to end, to the afferent vein graft stump at the time of loop division. Two AV loop cases (one Type 2, one Type 3) were connected to free flaps in a single stage, while the remaining case (Type 3) was performed in two stages to allow scheduling of a definitive free flap. In the two-stage AV loop, the arteriovenous fistula was left in place under skin flaps and then divided in a separate procedure six days later to allow for OR free flap scheduling.

Type 4 consisted of a Y shaped connection to recipient vessels, using vein graft branch points to supercharge flow to or from the flap. Type 4 vein graft case referenced in Table 1 (Patient E) involved arterial supercharging by connecting both the descending lateral femoral circumflex (DLFC) and the tensor fascia lata (TFL) pedicle arteries to branches of a Y shaped saphenous graft to cover a knee wound.

The diagrams in Figure 5 summarize the techniques used for anastomosis, expanding upon various vein graft patterns used for extending pedicle length to reliable vessels for free tissue transfer.

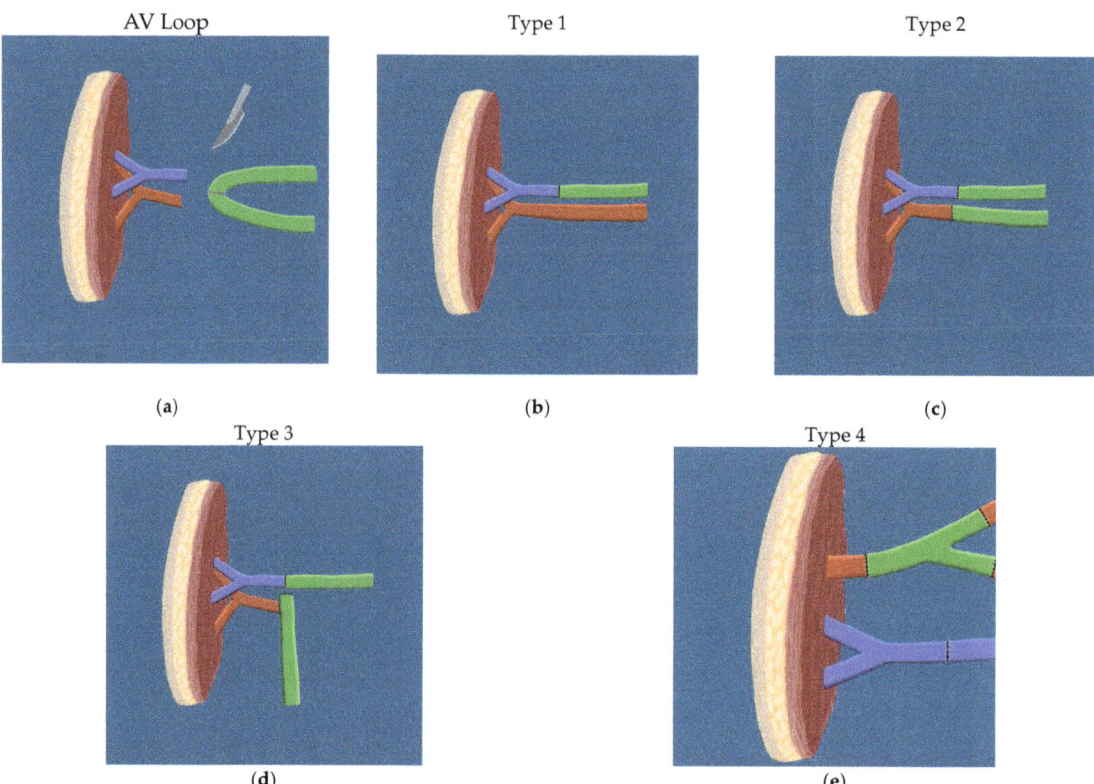

Figure 5. Illustrations showcasing various forms of anastomosis. (**a**) Initial AV loop creation, purple dotted line represents splitting of loop; (**b**) Type 1 end-to-end venous anastomosis; (**c**) Type 2, traditional AV loop anastomosis into vein and artery; (**d**) Type 3, mismatched AV loop with end-to-side arterial anastomosis with a stump. End-to-end venous anastomosis; (**e**) Type 4, arterial branch anastomosis allowing for increased arterial blood flow.

4. Discussion

This case series demonstrates the feasibility of massive flap reconstructions in heavily traumatized wounds using vein grafts as well as the reliability of these techniques across multiple surgeons. Three different surgeons at the same institution were involved in the care of these patients, and excellent outcomes were achieved in terms of flap viability, limb salvage, and amputation-free postoperative courses. Despite the increase in operative time required for vein graft harvest and vascular anastomosis, long segment vein grafting led to successful outcomes in this particular series. All patients exhibited dependable soft tissue healing and experienced successful follow-up, resulting in a 100% salvage rate and a 0% need for post-flap revision amputation. These outcomes compare favorably to the success rates reported in the established literature. Notably, Bost et al., Henn et al., Momeni et al., and Brumberg et al. all reported complex cases involving interpositional vein grafts and arteriovenous (AV) loops, with flap failure rates ranging from 3% to 20.3% [3–7]. Moreover, Lin et al., and Brumberg et al., who also explored limb salvage outcomes, reported impressive amputation-free survival rates of 83–93% and 90%, respectively [5–7]. In this practice, vein grafting was used in approximately 10% of free flap cases. In general, longer operative times were required for vein loop harvest cases compared to other free flap cases, but major venous thromboembolism was not encountered in any patients. Vein graft harvest itself adds approximately one to two hours of increased operative time for graft harvest and closure, as well as the need for additional microvascular anastomosis.

Takebacks or unplanned operations occurred in both acute and delayed post-operative phases. In the immediate post-operative period, venous thrombosis presented in the form of an expanding hematoma, which serves as a sentinel sign of venous compromise [8]. The existing literature underscores the importance of restoration and management of perfusion to ensure successful outcomes [9]. In both cases, mechanical causes were identified as reasons for the venous clot. The rate of re-exploration due to anastomotic causes was 20% in this small sample, a figure consistent with findings in prior literature. For instance, in Bos et al.'s series involving 90 interposition vein grafts and AV loops across 56 patients, 10 of the 42 vein-grafted flaps necessitated takeback for emergent salvage, with successful salvage achieved in 7 of these cases. In the same study, five two-stage vein grafts thrombosed before free flap transfer occurred [3]. Henn et al. presented a series of 103 cases involving arteriovenous loops, with observed thrombosis rates of 11–14%, major complication rates of 26–30%, and flap failure rates of 7–11% [4]. Lin et al. reported a case series encompassing 65 arteriovenous loops and interposition grafts for arterial pedicle elongation, revealing re-exploration rates ranging from 22% to 43% [5]. Additionally, Momeni et al. detailed one instance of re-exploration for arterial thrombosis in an AV loop case [6]. In this series, as in the case series referenced above, early re-exploration allowed for thrombectomy, excision of any damaged segment of vein graft, and clearance of any residual thrombus using tissue plasminogen activator drugs [10]. Additional experience, fluid resuscitation, and judicious use of chemoprophylaxis agents perioperatively could lead to a reduction in the incidence of these outcomes in future patients. One late, unplanned operation was performed for donor site seroma, a known complication of latissimus flap harvest. As additional cases were performed in the case series, the rate of unplanned takebacks decreased.

The outcomes and procedures in this case series are comparable to those in the established literature for vein or AV loop grafts for free tissue transfer. Bos et al. and Hen et al. presented a series of single- and two-stage AV loops with flap failure rates of 6%, and vein graft thrombectomy rates were reported to be higher for delayed two-stage AV loop cases [3,4]. Lin et al. presented a series of 65 cases of vein grafts longer than 20 cm for reconstruction and note re-exploration rates of 20–30% in select subgroups of cases [5]. In Momeni et al.'s series of 20 cases, outcomes for 10 AV-Loop free flaps were compared against 10 matched free flaps without vein grafts. Single-stage AV loop creation was found to have similar outcomes as those of free flaps that did not require vein grafting [6]. Brumberg et al. presented a series of 10 AV loop vein grafts for mangled lower extremity cases and noted amputation for infection in one case and 100% loop patency. In their series, AV loops were reported to be long, as corroborated by the practice of anastomosing loops to the popliteal and superficial femoral vessels for leg coverage [7]. The absence of thromboembolic events in our case series can be attributed to perioperative chemoprophylaxis use in this practice, but these data are not widely discussed in previous vein graft/free flap papers. While this practice is not universally implemented in reconstructive microsurgery cases, there is an increasing awareness of the importance of this clinical practice throughout plastic surgery [11].

In addition to reporting the reliability of these techniques, this case series demonstrates the versatility of vein grafts and highlights the feasibility of an end to side anastomosis to a stump on a vein graft. Four different vein graft constructs were implemented in this case series (Figure 5), and the use of vein grafts for venous pedicle extension was prevalent. While extending vein grafts to inflow pedicles remains a viable option, the collective experience of this group with extensive degloving and radiation injuries suggests that the quality of outflow vessels was comparatively less optimal (posing challenges in dissection due to fragility and small caliber) when compared to inflow vessels within the zone of injury. Vein grafting allowed for outflow to larger caliber veins in multiple instances. The use of vein grafts for venous pedicle extension alone is not widely represented in the literature, as most papers focus on arterial pedicle extension or AV loop creation.

Perhaps a common but under-reported practice among surgeons, arterial or venous supercharging can be accomplished using vein graft branch points (Figure 5, Type 4) [12]. In the one Type 4 case in this series, vasospasm was encountered along the DLFC system and TFL supercharging reliably improved flap perfusion and served as an adjunct to traditional vasospasm relieving techniques, such as use of topical calcium channel blockers, adventitial stripping, and warm heparinized saline irrigation. Similar practices are employed for augmenting venous outflow in the breast reconstruction along with head and neck literature to improve venous outflow [13,14].

In Figure 5, Type 3 AV loop patterns are noteworthy as a viable microsurgical salvage technique since neither case required anastomotic revision. The indication for this technique is a size mismatch between graft and flap arteries, a common phenomenon in saphenous loops connected to high inflow systems. In one case, a venotomy was required to directly sew the flap artery to the vein graft; a side branch of a vein graft was required in the other. The surgeons in this group reserved the Type 3 technique for inflow only, as a mismatch between thin, pliable veins may be more easily overcome compared to flap artery and vein graft size mismatches using traditional end-to-end anastomotic techniques. Venous vein graft segments demonstrate slower flow physiology than arterial vein graft limbs, which may increase the risk of venous thrombosis if there is turbulent flow within a stump adjacent to a venous anastomosis. In any case, an end-to-side arterial anastomosis to a stump of vein graft is a technique reported in the cardiac literature in cases of bypass grafting and should be employed if needed to complete the reconstruction. End-to-side and side-to-side anastomoses were demonstrated and juxtaposed as methods for linking small target coronary arteries to vein bypass grafts, with comparative analysis [15].

As acknowledged by multiple authors in the reconstructive literature, the thigh is an excellent reconstructive tissue bank [16]. The thigh donor site stood out as the predominant location utilized for flap harvesting. In general, dependable perforators are typically situated along the descending axis. In cases where the associated morbidity is considered acceptable, flaps derived from the tensor fasciae latae (TFL), vastus, or rectus muscles can serve as viable options [17]. When the wound size is relatively small in comparison to the extent of injury in the distal lower extremity, opting for the radial forearm flap can obviate the need for vein graft harvesting. Although a considerable amount of literature discusses the morbidity associated with the radial forearm flap, strategies for mitigating its impact have also been explored. Non-dominant forearm site harvest, use of an adipofascial flap design, placement of dermal regeneration templates over donor site flexor tendons, reconstruction of the radial artery and pre-operative and intraoperative pulse-oximetry Allen's testing have all led to acceptable outcomes in select patients [18]. Wounds with a large surface area of exposed critical structure can be covered with the latissimus flap, obviating the need for a vein graft [19]. The relatively larger surface area of this flap effectively lengthens the flap pedicle in addition to providing coverage of larger wounds. Nevertheless, in two instances within this series of latissimus flap procedures, vein graft augmentation was employed to extend the pedicle, underscoring the substantial magnitude of the degloving injuries observed in this particular case collection.

Even though saphenous veins were preferred as a source of grafts in this case series (90% of patients), deep vein or arterial grafts can be used when superficial veins are unusable or unavailable. The thigh tissue bank is also interesting because it can provide superficial, deep arterial, or venous grafts to elongate flap pedicle length [20]. As shown in case H, the venae comitantes of the descending lateral circumflex system can be used instead of saphenous grafts. In this manner, a second donor site can be avoided and reconstruction can be offered to patients with sclerosed or traumatized superficial veins, such as in cases of infection, degloving, or following venipuncture procedures. We found that the lumina of superficial veins are of adequate caliber to match to those of workhorse flap venae and are particularly useful when grafting is required for preserving outflow. That said, saphenous vein grafts are still the predominant source of vein grafts in the literature [21].

Several shortcomings of this data set should be acknowledged. The small sample size allows for the possibility that the reliability of vein grafting is not as high as reported in this case series of ten patients. However, the technical adaptability and remarkable success rates achieved within this cohort of patients showcases the efficacy of these methodologies, which, in terms of outcomes and intricacy, are on par with the literature on vein graft free flap procedures. Lin et al. reported an average vein graft length extension of 26–32 cm for elongating arterial pedicles, whereas in this study, the mean extension reached 37 cm [5]. Meanwhile, Brumberg et al. made reference to the use of long vein grafts in arteriovenous loops originating "at or above the knee" without specifying vein graft lengths [7]. This study also sheds light on the employment of vein grafts to supercharge arterial pedicles via branch points and successfully demonstrates end-to-side anastomosis with long segment vein grafts, both of which represent innovative arrangements that expand upon the established techniques of AV loop creation, which typically involves the creation of an arteriovenous fistula with end-to-end coaptations between the flap vessels and an interpositional vein graft [5,7]. Cavadas et al. presented a case involving bifurcated greater saphenous vein for double venous flow coaptation following AV loop creation, akin to the arterial supercharging seen in this series' Type 4 construct [22]. Moreover, the notably high proportion of vein grafts employed for extending venous pedicles (N = 5 in 10 cases) within this case series is a distinctive feature, as previous authors have predominantly described their use for either AV loop creation or arterial pedicle elongation [3–7]. While acknowledging the limitation of the small sample size in this case series, the 100% flap success rate and the absence of amputations among the associated patients, akin to the limb salvage rates in Lin et al. and Brumberg et al.'s vein graft series, provides compelling support for the utilization of these innovative techniques within this patient population. From that standpoint, this case series is valuable in the microsurgical vein graft literature. Another shortcoming of these data set is that operative time was not measured and could not be compared to matched cases without designing prospective databases on these cases. Besides expanding the number of patients in this series, future studies could focus on the morbidity of vein graft harvest, quantify wound measurements, compare operative time for vein graft harvest compared to matched cases, and detail long-term functionality of salvage patients using standardized protocols in this patient population [23,24].

Author Contributions: Conceptualization, B.C., K.K. and J.L.; methodology, K.K. and A.M.; software, T.R.; validation, B.C. and K.K.; formal analysis, B.C., K.K. and J.L. All authors have read and agreed to the published version of the manuscript.

Funding: This research received no external funding.

Institutional Review Board: The study was conducted according to the guidelines of the Declaration of Helsinki, and approved by the Institutional Review Board of Intermountain Health (ID: 1052396) (Approved and Accessed 9 August 2023).

Informed Consent Statement: Informed consent was obtained from all subjects involved in the study.

Data Availability Statement: The data presented in this study are available on request from the corresponding author. The data are not publicly available due to patient privacy.

Conflicts of Interest: The authors declare no conflict of interest.

References

1. Clarke-Pearson, E.M.; Kim, P.S. An effective method to access recipient vessels outside the zone of injury in free flap reconstruction of the lower extremity. *Ann. Plast. Surg.* **2014**, *73* (Suppl. S2), S136–S138. [CrossRef] [PubMed]
2. Loos, M.S.; Freeman, B.G.; Lorenzetti, A. Zone of injury: A critical review of the literature. *Ann. Plast. Surg.* **2010**, *65*, 573–577. [CrossRef] [PubMed]
3. Bos, T.J.B.; Calotta, N.A.; Seu, M.Y.B.; Cho, B.H.; Hassanein, A.H.M.M.; Rosson, G.D.; Cooney, D.S.; Sacks, J.M.M.M.F. Abstract QS13: Bridging The Gap: Extending Free Flap Pedicle Length With Interposition Vein Grafts And Arteriovenous Loops. *Plast. Reconstr. Surg.-Glob. Open* **2018**, *6*, 122. [CrossRef]
4. Henn, D.; Wähmann, M.S.T.; Horsch, M.; Hetjens, S.; Kremer, T.; Gazyakan, E.; Hirche, C.; Schmidt, V.J.; Germann, G.; Kneser, U. One-Stage versus Two-Stage Arteriovenous Loop Reconstructions: An Experience on 103 Cases from a Single Center. *Plast. Reconstr. Surg.* **2019**, *143*, 912–924. [CrossRef]
5. Lin, C.-H.; Mardini, S.; Lin, Y.-T.; Yeh, J.-T.; Wei, F.-C.; Chen, H.-C. Sixty-five clinical cases of free tissue transfer using long arteriovenous fistulas or vein grafts. *J. Trauma.* **2004**, *56*, 1107–1117. [CrossRef]
6. Momeni, A.; Lanni, M.A.; Levin, L.S.; Kovach, S.J. Does the use of arteriovenous loops increase complications rates in posttraumatic microsurgical lower extremity reconstruction?-A matched-pair analysis. *Microsurgery* **2018**, *38*, 605–610. [CrossRef]
7. Brumberg, R.S.; Kaelin, L.D.; Derosier, L.C.; Hutchinson, H. Early Results of Supporting Free Flap Coverage of Mangled Lower Extremities with Long Saphenous Arteriovenous Loop Grafts. *Ann. Vasc. Surg.* **2021**, *71*, 181–190. [CrossRef]
8. Yu, P.; Chang, D.W.; Miller, M.J.; Reece, G.; Robb, G.L. Analysis of 49 cases of flap compromise in 1310 free flaps for head and neck reconstruction. *Head Neck.* **2009**, *31*, 45–51. [CrossRef]
9. Coriddi, M.; Myers, P.; Mehrara, B.; Nelson, J.; Cordeiro, P.G.; Disa, J.; Matros, E.; Dayan, J.; Allen, R.; McCarthy, C. Management of postoperative microvascular compromise and ischemia reperfusion injury in breast reconstruction using autologous tissue transfer: Retrospective review of 2103 flaps. *Microsurgery* **2022**, *42*, 109–116. [CrossRef]
10. Serletti, J.M.; Moran, S.L.; Orlando, G.S.; O'connor, T.; Herrera, R.H. Urokinase protocol for free-flap salvage following prolonged venous thrombosis. *Plast. Reconstr. Surg.* **1998**, *102*, 1947–1953. [CrossRef]
11. Mirzamohammadi, F.; Silva, O.N.N.; Leaf, R.K.; Eberlin, K.R.; Valerio, I.L. Chemoprophylaxis and Management of Venous Thromboembolism in Microvascular Surgery. *Semin. Plast. Surg.* **2023**, *37*, 57–72. [CrossRef] [PubMed]
12. Tsao, C.K.; Chen, H.C.; Chen, H.T.; Coskunfirat, O.K. Using a Y-shaped vein graft with drain-out branches to provide additional arterial sources for free flap reconstruction in injured lower extremities. *Chang. Gung Med. J.* **2003**, *26*, 813–821. [PubMed]
13. Numajiri, T.; Sowa, Y.; Nishino, K.; Fujiwara, H.; Nakano, H.; Shimada, T.; Hisa, Y. Does a vascular supercharge improve the clinical outcome for free jejunal transfer? *Microsurgery* **2013**, *33*, 169–172. [CrossRef]
14. Chang, E.I.; Fearmonti, R.M.; Chang, D.W.; Butler, C.E. Cephalic Vein Transposition versus Vein Grafts for Venous Outflow in Free-flap Breast Reconstruction. *Plast. Reconstr. Surg. Glob. Open* **2014**, *2*, e141. [CrossRef]
15. Li, H.; Xie, B.; Gu, C.; Gao, M.; Zhang, F.; Wang, J.; Dai, L.; Yu, Y. Distal end side-to-side anastomoses of sequential vein graft to small target coronary arteries improve intraoperative graft flow. *BMC Cardiovasc. Disord.* **2014**, *14*, 65. [CrossRef] [PubMed]
16. Wong, C.-H.; Wei, F.-C. Anterolateral thigh flap. *Head Neck.* **2010**, *32*, 529–540. [CrossRef] [PubMed]
17. Posch, N.; Mureau, M.; Flood, S.; Hofer, S. The combined free partial vastus lateralis with anterolateral thigh perforator flap reconstruction of extensive composite defects. *Br. J. Plast. Surg.* **2005**, *58*, 1095–1103. [CrossRef]
18. Medina, M.; Salinas, H.M.; Eberlin, K.R.; Driscoll, D.N.; Kwon, J.Y.; Austen, W.; Cetrulo, C. Modified free radial forearm fascia flap reconstruction of lower extremity and foot wounds: Optimal contour and minimal donor-site morbidity. *J. Reconstr. Microsurg.* **2014**, *30*, 515–522. [CrossRef]
19. Kozusko, S.; Liu, X.; Riccio, C.; Chang, J.; Boyd, L.; Kokkalis, Z.; Konofaos, P. Selecting a free flap for soft tissue coverage in lower extremity reconstruction. *Injury* **2019**, *50* (Suppl. S5), S32–S39. [CrossRef]
20. Dorfman, D.W.; Pu, L.L. Using the descending branch of the lateral circumflex femoral artery and vein as recipient vessel for free tissue transfer to the difficult areas of the lower extremity. *Ann. Plast. Surg.* **2013**, *70*, 397–400. [CrossRef]
21. Vlastou, C.; Earle, A.S.; Jordan, R. Vein grafts in reconstructive microsurgery of the lower extremity. *Microsurgery* **1992**, *13*, 234–235. [CrossRef] [PubMed]
22. Cavadas, P.C.; Baklinska, M.; Almoguera-Martinez, A. Arteriovenous Vascular Loop Using a Bifurcated Greater Saphenous Vein. *Plast. Reconstr. Surg. Glob. Open* **2022**, *10*, e4036. [CrossRef] [PubMed]

23. Schirò, G.R.; Sessa, S.; Piccioli, A.; Maccauro, G. Primary amputation vs limb salvage in mangled extremity: A systematic review of the current scoring system. *BMC Musculoskelet. Disord.* **2015**, *16*, 372. [CrossRef] [PubMed]
24. Nayar, S.K.; Alcock, H.M.F.; Edwards, D.S. Primary amputation versus limb salvage in upper limb major trauma: A systematic review. *Eur. J. Orthop. Surg. Traumatol.* **2022**, *32*, 395–403. [CrossRef] [PubMed]

Disclaimer/Publisher's Note: The statements, opinions and data contained in all publications are solely those of the individual author(s) and contributor(s) and not of MDPI and/or the editor(s). MDPI and/or the editor(s) disclaim responsibility for any injury to people or property resulting from any ideas, methods, instructions or products referred to in the content.

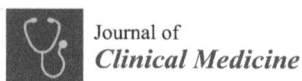 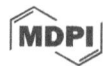

Article

Risk Factors for Flap Loss: Analysis of Donor and Recipient Vessel Morphology in Patients Undergoing Microvascular Head and Neck Reconstructions

Johannes G. Schuderer [1,*], Huong T. Dinh [1], Steffen Spoerl [1], Jürgen Taxis [1], Mathias Fiedler [1], Josef M. Gottsauner [1], Michael Maurer [1], Torsten E. Reichert [1], Johannes K. Meier [1], Florian Weber [2] and Tobias Ettl [1]

[1] Department of Oral and Maxillofacial Surgery, University Hospital Regensburg, 93053 Regensburg, Germany; juergen.taxis@ukr.de (J.T.); mathias1.fiedler@ukr.de (M.F.)
[2] Institute of Pathology, University Hospital Regensburg, 93053 Regensburg, Germany
* Correspondence: johannes.schuderer@ukr.de

Abstract: In microvascular head and neck reconstruction, various factors such as diabetes, alcohol consumption, and preoperative radiation hold a risk for flap loss. The primary objective of this study was to examine the vessel morphology of both recipient and donor vessels and to identify predictors for changes in the diameters of H.E.-stained specimens associated with flap loss in a prospective setting. Artery and vein samples (N = 191) were collected from patients (N = 100), with sampling from the recipient vessels in the neck area and the donor vessels prior to anastomosis. External vessel diameter transverse (ED), inner vessel diameter transverse (ID), thickness vessel intima (TI), thickness vessel media (TM), thickness vessel wall (TVW), and intima-media ratio (IMR) for the recipient (R) and transplant site (T) in arteries (A) and veins (V) were evaluated using H.E. staining. Flap loss (3%) was associated with increased ARED ($p = 0.004$) and ARID ($p = 0.004$). Preoperative radiotherapy led to a significant reduction in the outer diameter of the recipient vein in the neck ($p = 0.018$). Alcohol consumption ($p = 0.05$), previous thrombosis ($p = 0.007$), and diabetes ($p = 0.002$) were associated with an increase in the total thickness of venous recipient veins in the neck. Diabetes was also found to be associated with dilation of the venous media in the neck vessels ($p = 0.007$). The presence of cardiovascular disease (CVD) was associated with reduced intimal thickness ($p = 0.016$) and increased total venous vessel wall thickness ($p = 0.017$) at the transplant site. Revision surgeries were linked to increased internal and external diameters of the graft artery ($p = 0.04$ and $p = 0.003$, respectively), while patients with flap loss showed significantly increased artery diameters ($p = 0.004$). At the transplant site, alcohol influenced the enlargement of arm artery diameters ($p = 0.03$) and the intima–media ratio in the radial forearm flap ($p = 0.013$). In the anterolateral thigh, CVD significantly increased the intimal thickness and the intima–media ratio of the graft artery ($p = 0.01$ and $p = 0.02$, respectively). Patients with myocardial infarction displayed increased thickness in the *A. thyroidea* and artery media ($p = 0.003$). Facial arteries exhibited larger total vessel diameters in patients with CVD ($p = 0.03$), while facial arteries in patients with previous thrombosis had larger diameters and thicker media ($p = 0.01$). The presence of diabetes was associated with a reduced intima–media ratio ($p < 0.001$). Although the presence of diabetes, irradiation, and cardiovascular disease causes changes in vessel thickness in connecting vessels, these alterations did not adversely affect the overall success of the flap.

Keywords: microvascular reconstruction; free flap; flap loss; vessel anatomy; anastomosis

Citation: Schuderer, J.G.; Dinh, H.T.; Spoerl, S.; Taxis, J.; Fiedler, M.; Gottsauner, J.M.; Maurer, M.; Reichert, T.E.; Meier, J.K.; Weber, F.; et al. Risk Factors for Flap Loss: Analysis of Donor and Recipient Vessel Morphology in Patients Undergoing Microvascular Head and Neck Reconstructions. *J. Clin. Med.* 2023, *12*, 5206. https://doi.org/10.3390/jcm12165206

Academic Editors: Yves Harder and Emmanuel Andrès

Received: 22 June 2023
Revised: 26 July 2023
Accepted: 31 July 2023
Published: 10 August 2023
Corrected: 18 January 2024

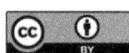

Copyright: © 2023 by the authors. Licensee MDPI, Basel, Switzerland. This article is an open access article distributed under the terms and conditions of the Creative Commons Attribution (CC BY) license (https://creativecommons.org/licenses/by/4.0/).

1. Introduction

Microvascular surgery is an established standard therapy for the functional rehabilitation of patients with defects in the head and neck region [1,2]. Microvascular grafts, such as the radial forearm flap (RFF) and the free fibula flap (FFF), facilitate the reconstruction of intricate defect scenarios by replacing multiple tissues in a single approach. Moreover, these grafts offer surgeons a sufficiently long vascular pedicle with a substantial vessel diameter [3,4]. Despite very good overall success rates of 95%, there are well-known factors that hold a risk of flap loss and seem to influence overall patient outcomes by compromising arterial and venous perfusion [5]. Smoking, alcohol consumption, and atherosclerosis have been shown to impact the success of microvascular reconstruction inducing histomorphologically apparent detrimental effects on vessels by causing endothelial dysfunction, chronic inflammation, and oxidative stress [6–9]. One additional common factor that seems to predict therapy setbacks is preoperative irradiation [5,10,11].

Upon histopathological examination, the morphology of free flap donor and recipient vessels in patients at risk show increased microscopic changes toward hyalinosis and inflammatory or prothrombotic features [12,13]. Next to changes in vessel wall diameters, changes in intima and media thickness in affected vessels are also presumed [14–16]. In addition, especially individuals with diabetes and arteriosclerosis may exhibit reduced vascular compliance, arterial stiffness, and impaired endothelial function, all of which can further impact the success of microvascular reconstruction by reducing local blood flow [17,18].

In this prospective study, we aimed to examine vessel morphology in both recipient and donor vessels and to identify predictors for changes in the diameters of H.E.-stained specimens. This may provide valuable insights into the impact of epidemiological factors on the success of microvascular reconstruction.

2. Material and Methods

All patients included in this study underwent ablative surgery and microvascular reconstruction due to neoplastic (tumor) or inflammatory diseases (osteomyelitis, necrosis) in the maxillofacial area at the Department of Oral and Maxillofacial Surgery. Both artery and vein samples were collected from the patient before anastomosis, with sampling from the recipient vessels in the neck area prior to suturing the graft. Samples of the donor vessels were taken from the pedicle immediately after graft harvest. Only vessels with intact integrity of the intima, media, and adventitia were submitted to pathology, while any vessels that were damaged or torn were excluded from the analysis.

The vascular specimens were fixed in 4% neutral buffered formalin in the operating theatre and transferred to the Institute of Pathology for complete formaldehyde fixation. Paraffin wax blocks were prepared using "ASP300S" (Leica Biosystems, Richmond, IL, USA) and "Histo Star" (Thermo Fisher Scientific, Schwerte, Germany). After cooling on the "PARA COOLER A" plate, the blocks were sectioned using the "Microm HM 340E with STS (Section Transfer System, Fisher Scientific, Schwerte, Germany)" rotary microtome and were mounted onto printed slides. The slides were then subjected to hematoxylin and eosin (HE) staining using "Histo Core SPECTRA ST" (Leica Biosystems, Richmond, IL, USA). All slides were digitally scanned using the Sysmex model "Panoramic 250 Flash III" (Sysmex, Norderstedt, Germany), and "Case Viewer" version 2.4 from the company 3D HISTECH Ltd (Budapest, Hungary). was used for microscopy and measurements.

Specific parameters were pre-defined to ensure consistency and reproducibility in measuring vessel diameter and stenosis in H.E. staining. The decision to measure these diameters was guided by the aim to maintain a straightforward examination under the microscope, encompassing external diameter, inner diameter, media and intima thickness, and total vessel wall thickness. For thickness and diameter measurements, a representative area of each vessel was carefully selected, excluding tangentially or only partially sectioned areas. A prior calibration of the measurement tool was conducted, and then the digital measurement tool was applied. Vessel examination was performed using a standardized $40\times$ magnification by a specialist in clinical pathology.

3. Patient Data

The records of patients who received microvascular flap reconstruction in this study were filtered. The patient data were evaluated, and a descriptive analysis was performed regarding epidemiological data, preoperative radiotherapy, nicotine and alcohol abuse, cardiovascular disease, and length of stay. Perioperative diagnoses were only included if they were ICD encoded in the discharge letter. In addition, tumor diagnosis or infectious states were recorded due to their ICD coding. With regard to microvascular reconstruction flap type, success and need for revision were documented.

From a prospective standpoint, flap success and flap revision were used as primary endpoints. In addition, the influence of the above-mentioned parameters on vessel wall thickness in H.E. staining was analyzed.

4. Statistics

Descriptive analyses were conducted in SPSS, and the variables were presented in absolute numbers and percentages. Univariate analyses were used to assess differences and correlations among the variables. The chi-squared test and t-test were used depending on the scale level and normal distribution of the compared variables. Statistical significance was set at $p < 0.05$. Vessel diameters were quantified in micrometers as the metric measurement unit. All analyses were conducted using SPSS version 26.0 (IBM Corp., Endicott, NY, USA).

5. Results

In this prospective study, we included 100 patients who received a microvascular graft for reconstruction in the head and neck region between 2021 and 2022.

The 100 patients consisted of 75 men and 25 women with a mean age of 65 ± 11.1 years. The patient population was divided into various diagnoses, including 63 oral squamous cell carcinomas, 17 cases of osteonecrosis of the jaw, 6 cases of osteomyelitis, and 6 cases of extraoral skin tumors. Eight patients underwent surgery and reconstruction for reasons such as trauma or salivary gland carcinomas. (Table 1).

Reconstruction was performed using various types of transplants, with free fibula flaps being the most frequently used (39%) followed by radial forearm flaps (37%). The mandible and floor of the mouth were the primary locations for reconstruction, accounting for 34% and 24% of cases, respectively. Other locations included the upper jaw (14%), tongue (9%), inner cheek (5%), and palate (5%). Nine cases required extraoral reconstruction, such as for the rehabilitation of the scalp after spinalioma resection.

The microvascular graft required revision in 6% of cases, and the overall success rate was 97%. The mean surgical time was 392 ± 104.2 min, with patients being hospitalized in the intensive care unit for an average of 4 ± 2.7 days and on the normal ward for 19 ± 9 days.

In terms of intraoperative vessels for microvascular anastomosis, the facial artery was selected for arterial anastomosis in 58% of cases, followed by the superficial thyroid artery (31%), the lingual artery (7%), and the superficial temporal artery (4%). For venous anastomosis, the facial vein was used in 47.3% of cases, the superficial thyroid vein in 35.5% of cases, the intrajugular vein in 10.7% of cases, and the external vein in 7.5% of cases. The superficial temporal vein was connected a total of four times.

In the retrospective patient evaluation, 34% of the patients had previously undergone head and neck radiotherapy, while 36% were documented to have nicotine abuse and 25% had alcohol abuse. A total of 10% of the patients had one or more thromboses prior to surgery, while 13% had experienced a myocardial infarction. In 27% of cases, cardiovascular disease was documented in the diagnoses of diabetes (14%). Detailed information is provided in Table 1.

The evaluation of vessel diameters using H.E. stain was conducted on a total of 70 transplant site arteries, 78 recipient site arteries, 13 transplant site veins, and 30 recipient site veins. Detailed results are provided in Table 2.

Table 1. Clinical characteristics regarding epidemiological and surgical features.

		N = 100	Revisions	p-Value	Flap Loss	p-Value
Sex	Male	75 (75%)	3		2	
	Female	25 (25%)	3		1	
Age	Years Ø	65 ± 11.1			61 ± 21.4	
Diagnosis				0.01		0.03
	OSCC	63 (63%)	1		-	
	Osteonecrosis of the jaw	17 (17%)	2		2	
	Osteomyelitis	6 (6%)	-		-	
	Cancer of skin	6 (6%)	2		1	
	Other	8 (8%)	1		-	
Flaps				0.9		0.9
	FFF	39 (39%)	3		2	
	RFF	37 (37%)	3		1	
	ALT	18 (18%)	-		-	
	Scapula	2 (2%)	-		-	
	Other	4 (4%)	-		-	
Localization				0.02		0.2
	Mandible	34 (34%)	3		2	
	Floor of the mouth	24 (24%)	0		-	
	Maxilla	14 (14%)	-		-	
	Tongue	9 (9%)	0		-	
	Planum buccale	5 (5%)	2		1	
	Palate	5 (5%)	-		-	
	Other	9 (9%)	1		-	
Flap Revision	Yes	6 (6%)	-		-	
Flap Loss	Yes	3 (3%)	-		-	
Operation time	Min Ø	392 ± 104.2	279 ± 162.8	0.003	221 ± 153.3	0.004
ICU	Days Ø	4 ± 2.7	3.7 ± 1.6	0.9	3 ± 1.7	0.2
NW	Days Ø	19 ± 9	22.4 ± 7	0.7	28 ± 5.1	0.1
Radiation	Yes	34 (34%)	2	0.9	2	0.2
Nicotine	Yes	36 (36%)	1	0.4	2	0.2
Alcohol	Yes	25 (25%)	2	0.6	2	0.1
s.p. Thrombosis	Yes	10 (10%)	1	0.5	-	0.7
s.p. MI	Yes	13 (13%)	1	0.2	-	0.4
CVD	Yes	27 (27%)	1	0.4	-	0.3
Diabetes	Yes	14 (14%)	2	0.3	1	0.2
Recipient artery						
	Facial	58 (58%)	4		2	
	Thyroidal sup.	31 (31%)	2		1	
	Lingual	7 (7%)	-		-	
	Temporal sup.	4 (4%)	-		-	
Recipient vein				0.001		0.002
	Facial	44 (47.3%)	4		1	
	Thyroidal sup	33 (35.5%)	-		-	
	Jugular interna	10 (10.7%)	-		-	
	Jugular externa	7 (7.5%)	2		2	
	Temporal sup.	4 (4.3%)	-		-	
	Other	2 (2.2%)	-		-	

CVD: cardiovascular disease; MI: myocardial infarction; ICU: intensive care unit; NW: normal ward; sup: superior; FFF: free fibula flap; RFF: radial forearm flap; ALT: anterior lateral thigh flap.

Table 2. Overall vessel morphology.

	AT	AR	VT	VR
N (191)	70	78	13	30
Diameter Ø	μm	μm	μm	μm
ED	2467.1 ± 549.4	2155.3 ± 515.6	2324.3 ± 683.5	2246.6 ± 663.4
ID	1456.3 ± 408.7	1216.6 ± 410.4	1554.8 ± 601.1	1433.5 ± 617.6
TI	115 ± 74	112 ± 84	32 ± 21	23 ± 16
TM	454 ± 148	407 ± 142	363 ± 160	368 ± 163
TVW	569 ± 181	519 ± 179	395 ± 161	391 ± 170
IMR	0.27 ± 0.19	0.29 ± 0.23	0.1 ± 0.07	0.68 ± 0.03
Hyalinosis	23	21	-	1

ED: external vessel diameter transverse; ID inner vessel diameter transverse; TI: thickness vessel intima; TM: thickness vessel media; TVW: thickness vessel wall; IMR: intima media ratio; AT: artery transplant site; AR: artery recipient site; VT: vein transplant site; VR: vein recipient site; μm: Vessel diameter in micrometers and mean value provided.

The univariate analyses showed that patients who received preoperative radiotherapy had a significant reduction in the outer diameter of the recipient vein in the neck (1966 μm vs. 2494 μm, respectively, $p = 0.018$). In addition, the total thickness of the venous recipient veins in the neck appeared to increase due to the influence of alcohol (519 μm vs. 360 μm, $p = 0.05$), previous thrombosis (505 μm vs. 389 μm, $p = 0.007$) and diabetes (476 μm vs. 396 μm, $p = 0.002$). The absolute thickness of the venous media in the neck vessels was significantly dilatated in the presence of diabetes (580 μm vs. 369 μm, $p = 0.007$). In addition, the presence of CVD led to a reduction in intimal thickness (1355 μm vs. 1613 μm, $p = 0.016$) and increased total venous vessel wall thickness (396 μm vs. 367 μm, $p = 0.017$) at the transplant site. A revision was significantly associated with an increased internal diameter of the graft artery (2018 μm vs. 1436 μm, $p = 0.04$) and increased external artery diameter at the neck (2667 μm vs. 2119 μm, $p = 0.003$). Patients with flap loss showed significantly increased vessel artery inner and outer diameter at the neck (3161 μm vs. 2120 μm, $p = 0.004$ resp. 2012 μm vs. 1188 μm, $p = 0.004$).

Breaking down the analyses by transplant revealed a significant enlargement in the outer diameter of arm arteries (2946 μm vs. 2604 μm, $p = 0.03$) and inner diameter (1690 μm vs. 1482 m, $p = 0.04$) under the influence of alcohol and an enlargement of the intima–media ratio of the vein in the RFF (0.14 vs. 0.09, $p = 0.013$). In ALT, CVD was shown to increase the intimal thickness (169 μm vs. 110 μm, $p = 0.01$) and the intima–media ratio of the graft artery (0.31 vs 0.30, $p = 0.02$) significantly. Fibula transplants were evaluated but did not show any association with the clinical parameters (Table 3).

Table 3. Flap site vessel diameters and associations with epidemiological factors in univariate analysis.

	ATED	ATID	ATTVW	ATTM	ATTI	ATIMR	VTED	VTID	VTTVW	VTTM	VTTI	VTIMR
RFF												
Ø in μm	2604.1	1482.2	642	498	144	0.30	2299.6	1414.8	488	454	34	0.09
Alcohol	2946.6 $p = 0.003$	1690.0 $p = 0.040$	693	544	149	0.29	2381.5	1249.5	602	571	29	0.06
CVD	2550.1	1441.3	671	540	130	0.24	2314.5	1516.5	425	374	54	0.14 $p = 0.03$
ALT												
Ø in μm	2593.3	1468.9	605	495	110	0.22	2730.5	1799.3	332	312	18	0.06
CVD	2656.0	1459.7	710	540	169 $p = 0.013$	0.31 $p = 0.020$						

RFF: radialis forearm flap; ALT: anterior lateral thigh flap; μm: vessel diameter in micrometers and median value provided; CVD: cardiovascular disease.

Univariate analyses also showed clinical differences in the individual vascular parameters regarding vessel type. In patients with myocardial infarction, the *A. thyroidea* as a recipient vessel showed an increase in the absolute vessel thickness (925 µm vs. 535 µm, $p = 0.003$) and an increase in the artery media thickness (701 µm vs. 413 µm, $p = 0.003$). Larger total vessel diameters (584 µm vs. 511 µm, $p = 0.03$) were measured for the facial artery in patients with CVD. Recipient facial arteries from patients with previous thrombosis were also larger (672 µm vs. 511 µm, $p = 0.01$) and had a thicker media (512 µm vs. 395 µm, $p = 0.01$). Finally, specimens with the presence of diabetes had a significantly reduced intima–media ratio (0.13 vs. 0.32, $p < 0.001$).

In terms of radiation, the *A. facialis* showed a significantly lower intern diameter (1246 µm vs 1149 µm, $p = 0.04$) and a smaller intima (116 µm vs. 144.5 µm, $p = 0.01$) with a reduced intima–media ratio (0.3 vs 0.32, $p = 0.02$). The temporal artery showed significantly lower total vessel wall thickness (296.6 µm vs. 876 µm, $p = 0.04$) and reduced media thickness (235.5 µm vs. 790 µm, $p = 0.02$). The IMR was increased (0.24 vs 0.11, $p = 0.01$) (Figure 1).

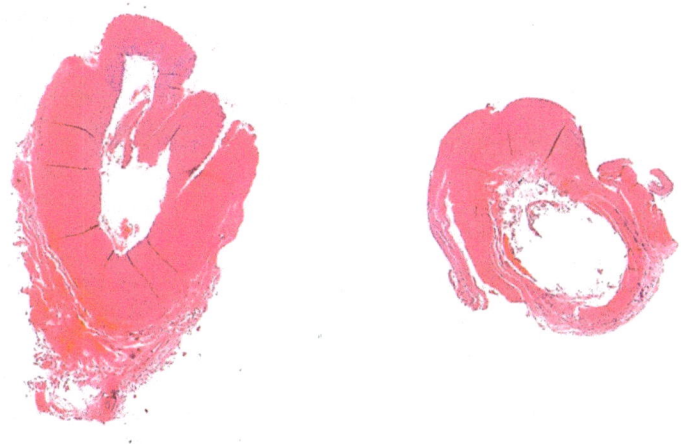

Figure 1. Recipient temporal superficial artery (**left**) without and (**right**) with pre radiotherapy H.E. staining, 40× zoom.

In the case of facial venous connecting vessels, alcohol had an influence on the thickness of the vein (472 µm vs. 388 µm, $p = 0.038$) and the media thickness (452 µm vs. 366 µm, $p = 0.035$). Diabetes increased vessel thickness (592 µm vs. 388 µm, $p = 0.027$) and media thickness (577 µm vs. 366 µm, $p = 0.022$), respectively. In addition, the intima–media ratio appeared to be reduced (0.02 vs 0.07, $p < 0.001$). Regarding the internal jugular vein, nicotine (20 µm vs. 15 µm, $p = 0.002$) and CVD (12 µm vs. 15 µm, $p = 0.002$) each lead to a reciprocal change in intimal thickness (Table 4).

Table 4. Recipient vessel diameters and associations with epidemiological factors in univariate analysis.

	ARED	ARID	ARTVW	ARTM	ARTI	ARIMR
A. thyroidea superior						
Ø in µm	2107.7	1197.7	535	413	122	0.32
MI	2584.3	1102.8	925 $p = 0.003$	701 $p = 0.003$	224	0.32

Table 4. Cont.

	ARED	ARID	ARTVW	ARTM	ARTI	ARIMR
A. facialis						
Ø in μm	2216.7	1246.4	511	395	116	0.31
CVD	2255.2	1134.3	584 $p = 0.037$	425	158	0.36
Thrombosis	2616,6 $p < 0.001$	1471.4	672 $p = 0.016$	512 $p = 0.011$	161	0.33
Diabetes	2104.3	1250.6	487	429	59	0.13 $p < 0.001$
Radiation	20589	1149.3 $p = 0.04$	552.8	436.7	114.8 $p = 0.01$	0.30 $p = 0.02$
A. Temporalis						
Ø in μm	2067.5	1158	876	790	89	0.11
Radiation	1418.2	862	296.6 $p = 0.04$	235.5 $p = 0.02$	55.5	0.24 $p = 0.01$
	VRED	VRID	VRTVW	VRTM	VRTI	VRIMR
V. facialis						
Ø in μm	2360.0	1563.7	388	366	21	0.07
Alcohol	2198.3	1242.8	472 $p = 0.038$	452 $p = 0.035$	20	0.06
Diabetes	2283.5	1394.3	592 $p = 0.027$	577 $p = 0.022$	15	0.02 $p < 0.001$
Radiation	1943.8 $p = 0.44$	1334.8	335	337.5	16.25	0.08
V. jugularis interna						
Ø in μm	2012.3	1177.3	383	369	15	0.04
Nicotine	2270.8	1035.8	398	382	20 $p = 0.002$	0.05
CVD	1840	1271.7	373	360	12 $p = 0.002$	0.04

A: artery; V: vein; μm: vessel diameter in micrometers and median value provided; CVD: cardiovascular disease.

6. Discussion

In general, the reconstruction of head and neck defects using free microvascular transplants represents an essential aspect of routine clinical practice. The growing proportion of older and medically complex patients presents clinical challenges during the procedural planning phase. Accurate preoperative visualization of vessels is critical, especially in flap preparation, as observed in the case of free fibula flap (FFF). However, challenges during anastomosis unrelated to the flap's macroscopic characteristics may emerge, potentially resulting in immediate revision or flap loss. [19]. Pries and colleagues demonstrated the influence of both local and systemic stress on the adaptive capacity of peripheral and central vessels, revealing that vessel wall thickness adapts to both mechanical and metabolic stimuli [20].

In our investigation, we examined the impact of diverse patient-related factors on the morphology of both the donor and recipient vessels in H.E. staining and their correlation with the outcome of flap success or revision.

In general, the need for transplant revision or flap loss appears to be multifactorial. One important factor is vessel quality and morphology during anastomosis. Traditionally, thrombosis in the vein or artery leads to congestion or reduced blood flow, manifested as a discoloration of the transplant and poor intraoperative perfusion. In our study, a total of 6% of the flaps were revised with an overall success of 97%. This is consistent with data on success rates in the literature [5,11].

An important factor that has been subject to controversial discussions in the literature is the impact of radiation on the vascular morphology of neck vessels, directly influencing the success of graft procedures. [10]. In a comprehensive study involving over 850 participants, Tan et al. failed to demonstrate any significant effect of preoperative irradiation on the success of microvascular reconstruction [21]. However, in a meta-analysis conducted by Mijiti et al., a pooled odds ratio (OR) of 1.82 was reported for flap loss in association with preoperative irradiation. [10].

In our study, the presence of preoperative irradiation was significantly associated with a reduction in the thickness of the recipient vein ($p = 0.018$) but was not associated with overall flap success. From a clinical point of view, this result corresponds to the increased risk of venous injury during the preparation of the venous recipient vessel. In further subgroup analyses, a significant reduction in the intima and media thickness was observed in A. and V. facialis and A. temporalis. (Table 3, Figure 1). In the context of the calvaria and lower jaw, the development of osteoradionecrosis (IORN) in the cranial and mandible vault following radiation therapy for local tumor control is not uncommon [22,23]. Subsequently, the connection of microvascular grafts via the temporal or facial vascular axis becomes necessary. However, flap success in the pre-irradiated area poses a significant challenge [24]. Shonka and colleagues conducted a study involving 62 microvascular scalp reconstructions, revealing that 89% of the reported complications occurred specifically within the pre-irradiated tissue region [25]. In their study, Hirsch et al. reported a marginal decrease in the flap success rate of 88% among patients undergoing mandibular reconstruction for osteoradionecrosis. Nevertheless, no statistically significant disparities were observed when compared to the primary tumor reconstruction group [26].

Preidl et al. explicated the mechanisms underlying vascular changes subsequent to radiotherapy in patients, unveiling the emergence of prothrombotic and inflammatory alterations that precipitate endothelial dysfunction [14]. It is plausible to posit that common factors, such as irradiation and high blood pressure, can reduce vascular vasodilation, which in turn disrupts the balance between the pro- and antithrombotic activity of the endothelium, as reported by Rajendran et al. in 2013 [27]. Despite this, microvascular reconstruction appears to be a safe and feasible option for patients with osteoradionecrosis of the jaw or scalp, with no significant decrease in success rates, according to a study by Sweeny et al. in 2021 [23].

Patients who underwent revision exhibited a significant increase in inner (ATID, $p = 0.04$) and external (ARED, $p = 0.03$) vessel diameter of the transplant artery upon microscopic examination. Moreover, the presence of flap loss was associated with a significant increase in the outer and inner diameters of the recipient neck arteries compared to the rest of the patient population ($p = 0.004$). These findings should be considered in the context of the overall results. Notably, alcohol abuse, a history of thrombosis, cardiovascular disease (CVD), and diabetes were all associated with increased thickness of vessel segments. In particular, a direct correlation between these factors and an increase in overall vessel wall thickness of recipient veins in the neck was observed ($p = 0.03$) (see Table 5).

Table 5. Correlations between vessel diameter and patient characteristics identified using univariate analyses.

Ø in μm		ATID	ATED	ATTM	ARID	ARED	ARTM	ARTVW	VTVW	VTTI	VRID	VRED	VRTM	VRTVW
Sex			$p = 0.03$											
	M		2530.2 ± 28.4											
	F		2217.6 ± 533.1											
Radiation					$p = 0.034$						$p = 0.03$	$p = 0.018$		
	y				92.25 ± 55						1229.9 ± 341	1966.042 ± 343.3919		
	n				123.38 ± 95.3						1605 ± 716	2494.278 ± 714.0903		
Alcohol			$p = 0.005$	$p = 0.03$										$p = 0.05$
	y		2716.6 ± 372.8	517.28 ± 157.585										519.00 ± 101.628
	n		2363.5 ± 565.2	431.04 ± 140.707										360.70 ± 169.153
TE							$p = 0.016$	$p = 0.024$						$p = 0.007$
	y						539.75 ± 204.072	657.75 ± 223.713						505.50 ± 149.200
	n						390.76 ± 127.343	502.58 ± 169.848						389.93 ± 169.830
CVD									$p = 0.017$	$p = 0.016$				
	y								396.00 ± 56.107	1355.833 ± 344.4566				
	n								367.10 ± 166.786	1613.850 ± 691.7320				
Diabetes								$p = 0.009$					$p = 0.007$	$p = 0.002$
	y							546.33 ± 178.079					580.50 ± 64.568	476.56 ± 159.931
	n							514.52 ± 181.664					369.50 ± 162.369	396.68 ± 138.723
Revision		$p = 0.04$				$p = 0.03$								
	y	2018.75 ± 35.7				2667 ± 815								
	n	14346 ± 403.5				2119.3 ± 484								
Flap loss					$p = 0.004$	$p = 0.004$								
	y				2012.2 ± 488	3161 ± 847.8								
	n				1188.1 ± 385	2120.7 ± 482								

ATID: artery transplant internal diameter (μm); ATED: artery transplant external diameter (μm); ATTM: artery transplant total media thickness (μm); ARID: artery recipient site internal diameter (μm); ARED: artery recipient vessel external diameter (μm); ARTM: artery recipient site total media thickness (μm); ARTVW: artery recipient site total vessel wall thickness (μm); VTVW: vein transplant total vessel wall thickness (μm); VTTI: vein transplant total intima thickness (μm); VRID: vein recipient site internal diameter (μm); VRED: vein recipient site external diameter (μm); VRTM: vein recipient site total media thickness (μm); VRTVW: vein recipient site total vessel wall thickness (μm); TE: condition after thromboembolism, CVD: cardiovascular disease; μm: vessel diameter in micrometers and mean value provided.

The presence of diabetes was associated with a significant increase in venous media enlargement ($p = 0.007$). Moreover, the analysis based on adjacent vessels revealed a noteworthy decrease in the intima-to-media ratio for both the facial artery (ARIMR: $p < 0.001$) and facial vein (VRIMR: $p < 0.001$) at the anastomosis site. According to Ueno et al. (2021), vessel wall thickness increases in patients with diabetes, which ultimately leads to impaired arterial blood flow [16]. The mechanisms underlying this phenomenon include hypertension with initial hyperperfusion and subsequent endothelial dysfunction, resulting in the expression of endothelin-1 and angiotensin II, ultimately leading to the remodeling of vascular anatomy with hypertrophy and fibrosis [28,29]. Valentini et al. were able to describe diabetes from various risk factors as a clear independent predictor for a worse flap outcome [30].

Moreover, there is a noticeable association between thrombosis and an increase in wall and media thickness in both the arteries and veins located in the neck ($p = 0.007$, $p = 0.016$, $p = 0.024$). The plausibility of the relationship between a history of thrombosis and changes in the morphology of vessels in the extremities or neck is evident. As per Falanga et al., cancer patients exhibit an imbalance in the hemostatic system that makes them up to seven times more vulnerable to thrombosis [31]. This hypercoagulable state arises from both direct and indirect mechanisms, resulting in the formation of thrombi [32]. Furthermore, there is evidence to suggest a long-term alteration of the patient's vessels through the expression of metalloproteinases and subsequent vascular remodeling [33]. However, it is important to note that the risk of developing thrombosis and changes in vessel morphology in the extremities and neck share similar risk factors, including age, diabetes, and cardiovascular disease, as well as prior chemotherapy, radiation therapy, or medication use [32].

Our analysis suggests a discernible impact of long-term alcohol abuse on both the flap and neck vessel sites. Specifically, the outer diameter of the arterial vessel ($p = 0.05$) and the media ($p = 0.03$) flap site appeared to be significantly thickened ($p = 0.005$). Moreover, the entire vessel wall of the recipient vein was observed to be thickened as well ($p = 0.05$). Remarkably, in the sub-analysis, the same effects in the RFF ($p = 0.03$) and facial vein ($p = 0.03$) were observed. The influence of long-term alcohol consumption on vascular anatomy is multifaceted, with ethanol exerting both vascular and central effects on various regulatory axes, such as intracellular calcium levels and NO regulation, which may modulate vasodilation [34,35]. Additionally, the renin–angiotensin–aldosterone system (RAAS) is involved, resulting in elevated blood pressure [34], which together finally leads to atherosclerosis [36]. Hence, all the factors mentioned above not only contribute to the deterioration of the patient's overall health, thereby elevating the risk of postoperative nosocomial complications, but also directly induce visible alterations in the vessels. These changes may pose challenges for surgeons during anastomosis, even under optimal conditions. Therefore, it becomes imperative to acknowledge and address these factors proactively for better surgical outcomes in the future.

This study has certain limitations. Despite its prospective design, the histopathologic examination of vessel gating may be susceptible to potential errors. Alongside the possibility of erroneous staining, there exists a potential concern that the chosen sections might not be entirely representative, thereby potentially leading to over- or underestimation of the corresponding vessel diameters. To bolster these aspects, the incorporation of immunohistochemical techniques could provide additional support and reliability to the findings.

7. Conclusions

In conclusion, our study revealed significant associations between vascular parameters in the context of flap loss, preoperative radiotherapy, alcohol consumption, previous thrombosis, diabetes, cardiovascular disease (CVD), revision surgeries, and myocardial infarction. Flap loss was linked to increased arteriolar diameters and vein thickness, while preoperative radiotherapy led to a reduced outer diameter of the recipient veins. Alcohol consumption, previous thrombosis, and diabetes were associated with increased total thickness of venous recipient veins, with diabetes also showing venous media dilation. The presence of CVD was related to reduced intimal thickness and increased total vessel wall thickness at the transplant site. Though microvascular reconstruction seems safe even in a complex patient clientele, our findings shed light on the intricate interplay between various factors and vascular parameters, providing valuable insights for clinical practice and further research in reconstructive surgery.

Author Contributions: Conceptualization: J.G.S., F.W. and T.E.; data curation, H.T.D., J.M.G. and J.K.M.; formal analysis, J.G.S., H.T.D., M.M. and J.K.M.; investigation, F.W.; methodology, J.T., M.F., J.M.G. and T.E.; project administration, T.E.R.; resources, S.S., J.T. and T.E.R.; software, M.F., J.K.M. and F.W.; supervision, S.S. and T.E.; visualization, M.M. and F.W.; writing—original draft, J.G.S.; writing—review and editing, T.E. All authors have read and agreed to the published version of the manuscript.

Funding: This research received no external funding.

Institutional Review Board Statement: This study was conducted under local ethical committee approval (Nr: 18-1131-104) and conducted in accordance with ethical standards of the Declaration of Helsinki.

Informed Consent Statement: Signing informed consent was not required based on the conducted analysis, the fully anonymized set of clinical data, and in accordance with the Ethics Committee's decision.

Data Availability Statement: The data can be obtained by scientists that conduct work independently from the industry, on request. The data are not stored on publicly available servers.

Conflicts of Interest: The authors declare no conflict of interest.

References

1. Meier, J.K.; Schuderer, J.G.; Zeman, F.; Klingelhöffer, C.; Hullmann, M.; Spanier, G.; Reichert, T.E.; Ettl, T. Health-related quality of life: A retrospective study on local vs. microvascular reconstruction in patients with oral cancer. *BMC Oral Health* **2019**, *19*, 62. [CrossRef]
2. Pohlenz, P.; Klatt, J.; Schön, G.; Blessmann, M.; Li, L.; Schmelzle, R. Microvascular free flaps in head and neck surgery: Complications and outcome of 1000 flaps. *Int. J. Oral Maxillofac. Surg.* **2012**, *41*, 739–743. [CrossRef] [PubMed]
3. Ettl, T.; Gottsauner, M.; Kühnel, T.; Maurer, M.; Schuderer, J.G.; Spörl, S.; Taxis, J.; Reichert, T.E.; Fiedler, M.; Meier, J.K. The Folded Radial Forearm Flap in Lip and Nose Reconstruction—Still a Unique Choice. *J. Clin. Med.* **2023**, *12*, 3636. [CrossRef] [PubMed]
4. Schuderer, J.G.; Meier, J.K.; Klingelhöffer, C.; Gottsauner, M.; Reichert, T.E.; Wendl, C.M.; Ettl, T. Magnetic resonance angiography for free fibula harvest: Anatomy and perforator mapping. *Int. J. Oral Maxillofac. Surg.* **2019**, *49*, 176–182. [CrossRef]
5. Zhou, W.; Zhang, W.-B.; Yu, Y.; Wang, Y.; Mao, C.; Guo, C.-B.; Yu, G.-Y.; Peng, X. Risk factors for free flap failure: A retrospective analysis of 881 free flaps for head and neck defect reconstruction. *Int. J. Oral Maxillofac. Surg.* **2017**, *46*, 941–945. [CrossRef]
6. Garip, M.; Van Dessel, J.; Grosjean, L.; Politis, C.; Bila, M. The impact of smoking on surgical complications after head and neck reconstructive surgery with a free vascularised tissue flap: A systematic review and meta-analysis. *Br. J. Oral Maxillofac. Surgery* **2021**, *59*, e79–e98. [CrossRef]
7. Lee, M.K.; Blackwell, K.E.; Kim, B.; Nabili, V. Feasibility of Microvascular Head and Neck Reconstruction in the Setting of Calcified Arteriosclerosis of the Vascular Pedicle. *JAMA Facial Plast. Surg.* **2013**, *15*, 135. [CrossRef]
8. Phillips, S.A.; Osborn, K.; Hwang, C.-L.; Sabbahi, A.; Piano, M.R. Ethanol induced oxidative stress in the vasculature: Friend or Foe. *Curr. Hypertens. Rev.* **2020**, *16*, 181–191. [CrossRef] [PubMed]
9. Rosado, P.; Cheng, H.-T.; Wu, C.-M.; Wei, F.-C. Influence of diabetes mellitus on postoperative complications and failure in head and neck free flap reconstruction: A systematic review and meta-analysis. *Head Neck* **2015**, *37*, 615–618. [CrossRef]
10. Mijiti, A.; Kuerbantayi, N.; Zhang, Z.Q.; Su, M.Y.; Zhang, X.H.; Huojia, M. Influence of preoperative radiotherapy on head and neck free-flap reconstruction: Systematic review and meta-analysis. *Head Neck* **2020**, *42*, 2165–2180. [CrossRef]
11. Preidl, R.H.M.; Wehrhan, F.; Schlittenbauer, T.; Neukam, F.W.; Stockmann, P. Perioperative factors that influence the outcome of microsurgical reconstructions in craniomaxillofacial surgery. *Br. J. Oral Maxillofac. Surg.* **2015**, *53*, 533–537. [CrossRef]
12. Preidl, R.H.M.; Möbius, P.; Weber, M.; Amann, K.; Neukam, F.W.; Schlegel, A.; Wehrhan, F. Expression of transforming growth factor beta 1-related signaling proteins in irradiated vessels. *Strahlenther. Onkol.* **2015**, *191*, 518–524. [CrossRef] [PubMed]

13. Schultze-Mosgau, S.; Erbe, M.; Keilholz, L.; Radespiel-Tröger, M.; Wiltfang, J.; Minge, N.; Neukam, F.W. Histomorphometric analysis of irradiated recipient vessels and transplant vessels of free flaps in patients undergoing reconstruction after ablative surgery. *Int. J. Oral Maxillofac. Surg.* **2000**, *29*, 112–118. [CrossRef] [PubMed]
14. Preidl, R.H.M.; Möbius, P.; Weber, M.; Amann, K.; Neukam, F.W.; Kesting, M.; Geppert, C.-I.; Wehrhan, F. Long-term endothelial dysfunction in irradiated vessels: An immunohistochemical analysis. *Strahlenther. Onkol.* **2019**, *195*, 52–61. [CrossRef] [PubMed]
15. Tall, J.; Björklund, T.; Skogh, A.-C.; Arnander, C.; Halle, M. Vascular Complications After Radiotherapy in Head and Neck Free Flap Reconstruction: Clinical Outcome Related to Vascular Biology. *Ann. Plast. Surg.* **2015**, *75*, 309–315. [CrossRef]
16. Ueno, Y.; Iwase, T.; Goto, K.; Tomita, R.; Ra, E.; Yamamoto, K.; Terasaki, H. Association of changes of retinal vessels diameter with ocular blood flow in eyes with diabetic retinopathy. *Sci. Rep.* **2021**, *11*, 4653. [CrossRef]
17. de Bree, R.; Quak, J.J.; Kummer, J.A.; Simsek, S.; Leemans, C.R. Severe atherosclerosis of the radial artery in a free radial forearm flap precluding its use. *Oral Oncol.* **2004**, *40*, 99–102. [CrossRef]
18. Lese, I.; Biedermann, R.; Constantinescu, M.; Grobbelaar, A.O.; Olariu, R. Predicting risk factors that lead to free flap failure and vascular compromise: A single unit experience with 565 free tissue transfers. *J. Plast. Reconstr. Aesthetic Surg.* **2021**, *74*, 512–522. [CrossRef]
19. Preidl, R.H.M.; Reuss, S.; Neukam, F.W.; Kesting, M.; Wehrhan, F. Endothelial inflammatory and thrombogenic expression changes in microvascular anastomoses—An immunohistochemical analysis. *J. Cranio-Maxillofac. Surg.* **2021**, *49*, 422–429. [CrossRef]
20. Pries, A.R.; Reglin, B.; Secomb, T.W. Remodeling of Blood Vessels. *Hypertension* **2005**, *46*, 725–731. [CrossRef]
21. Tan, N.C.; Lin, P.-Y.; Chiang, Y.-C.; Chew, K.-Y.; Chen, C.-C.; Fujiwara, T.; Kuo, Y.-R. Influence of neck dissection and preoperative irradiation on microvascular head and neck reconstruction—Analysis of 853 cases. *Microsurgery* **2014**, *34*, 602–607. [CrossRef] [PubMed]
22. Lee, M.; Chin, R.Y.; Eslick, G.D.; Sritharan, N.; Paramaesvaran, S. Outcomes of microvascular free flap reconstruction for mandibular osteoradionecrosis: A systematic review. *J. Cranio-Maxillofac. Surg.* **2015**, *43*, 2026–2033. [CrossRef] [PubMed]
23. Sweeny, L.; Mayland, E.; Swendseid, B.P.; Curry, J.M.; Kejner, A.E.; Thomas, C.M.; Kain, J.J.; Cannady, S.B.; Tasche, K.; Rosenthal, E.L.; et al. Microvascular Reconstruction of Osteonecrosis: Assessment of Long-term Quality of Life. *Otolaryngol. Head Neck Surg.* **2021**, *165*, 636–646. [CrossRef] [PubMed]
24. Schuderer, J.G.; Spörl, S.; Spanier, G.; Gottsauner, M.; Gessner, A.; Hitzenbichler, F.; Meier, J.; Reichert, T.E.; Ettl, T. Surgical and remote site infections after reconstructive surgery of the head and neck: A risk factor analysis. *J. Cranio-Maxillofac. Surg.* **2022**, *50*, 178–187. [CrossRef]
25. Shonka, D.C.; Potash, A.E.; Jameson, M.J.; Funk, G.F. Successful reconstruction of scalp and skull defects: Lessons learned from a large series: Successful Reconstruction of Scalp and Skull Defects. *Laryngoscope* **2011**, *121*, 2305–2312. [CrossRef]
26. Hirsch, D.L.; Bell, R.B.; Dierks, E.J.; Potter, J.K.; Potter, B.E. Analysis of Microvascular Free Flaps for Reconstruction of Advanced Mandibular Osteoradionecrosis: A Retrospective Cohort Study. *J. Oral Maxillofac. Surg.* **2008**, *66*, 2545–2556. [CrossRef]
27. Rajendran, P.; Rengarajan, T.; Thangavel, J.; Nishigaki, Y.; Sakthisekaran, D.; Sethi, G.; Nishigaki, I. The Vascular Endothelium and Human Diseases. *Int. J. Biol. Sci.* **2013**, *9*, 1057–1069. [CrossRef]
28. Intengan, H.D.; Schiffrin, E.L. Vascular Remodeling in Hypertension. *Hypertension* **2012**, *59*, 367–374. [CrossRef]
29. Schiffrin, E. Remodeling of resistance arteries in essential hypertension and effects of antihypertensive treatment. *Am. J. Hypertens.* **2004**, *17*, 1192–1200. [CrossRef]
30. Valentini, V.; Cassoni, A.; Marianetti, T.M.; Mitro, V.; Gennaro, P.; Ialongo, C.; Iannetti, G. Diabetes as Main Risk Factor in Head and Neck Reconstructive Surgery With Free Flaps. *J. Craniofacial Surg.* **2008**, *19*, 1080. [CrossRef]
31. Falanga, A.; Russo, L.; Milesi, V.; Vignoli, A. Mechanisms and risk factors of thrombosis in cancer. *Crit. Rev. Oncol./Hematol.* **2017**, *118*, 79–83. [CrossRef] [PubMed]
32. Abdol Razak, N.B.; Jones, G.; Bhandari, M.; Berndt, M.C.; Metharom, P. Cancer-Associated Thrombosis: An Overview of Mechanisms, Risk Factors, and Treatment. *Cancers* **2018**, *10*, 380. [CrossRef]
33. Deatrick, K.B.; Elfline, M.; Baker, N.; Luke, C.E.; Blackburn, S.; Stabler, C.; Wakefield, T.W.; Henke, P.K. Postthrombotic vein wall remodeling: Preliminary observations. *J. Vasc. Surg.* **2011**, *53*, 139–146. [CrossRef]
34. Marchi, K.C.; Muniz, J.J.; Tirapelli, C.R. Hypertension and chronic ethanol consumption: What do we know after a century of study? *World J. Cardiol.* **2014**, *6*, 283–294. [CrossRef] [PubMed]
35. Piano, M.R. Alcohol's Effects on the Cardiovascular System. *Alcohol Res.* **2017**, *38*, 219–241.
36. Teragawa, H.; Fukuda, Y.; Matsuda, K.; Higashi, Y.; Yamagata, T.; Matsuura, H.; Chayama, K. Effect of alcohol consumption on endothelial function in men with coronary artery disease. *Atherosclerosis* **2002**, *165*, 145–152. [CrossRef] [PubMed]

Disclaimer/Publisher's Note: The statements, opinions and data contained in all publications are solely those of the individual author(s) and contributor(s) and not of MDPI and/or the editor(s). MDPI and/or the editor(s) disclaim responsibility for any injury to people or property resulting from any ideas, methods, instructions or products referred to in the content.

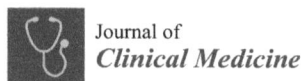 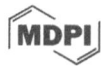

Systematic Review

The Expanding Utility of Robotic-Assisted Flap Harvest in Autologous Breast Reconstruction: A Systematic Review

Nikita Roy [1], Christopher J. Alessandro [2], Taylor J. Ibelli [1], Arya A. Akhavan [1], Jake M. Sharaf [1], David Rabinovitch [3], Peter W. Henderson [1] and Alice Yao [1,*]

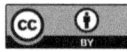

Citation: Roy, N.; Alessandro, C.J.; Ibelli, T.J.; Akhavan, A.A.; Sharaf, J.M.; Rabinovitch, D.; Henderson, P.W.; Yao, A. The Expanding Utility of Robotic-Assisted Flap Harvest in Autologous Breast Reconstruction: A Systematic Review. *J. Clin. Med.* **2023**, *12*, 4951. https://doi.org/10.3390/jcm12154951

Academic Editor: Salvatore Giordano

Received: 26 May 2023
Revised: 22 June 2023
Accepted: 27 June 2023
Published: 27 July 2023

Copyright: © 2023 by the authors. Licensee MDPI, Basel, Switzerland. This article is an open access article distributed under the terms and conditions of the Creative Commons Attribution (CC BY) license (https://creativecommons.org/licenses/by/4.0/).

[1] Division of Plastic and Reconstructive Surgery, Department of Surgery, Icahn School of Medicine at Mount Sinai, New York, NY 10029, USA; nikita.roy@icahn.mssm.edu (N.R.); taylor.ibelli@gmail.com (T.J.I.); akhavan.andre.arya@gmail.com (A.A.A.); jmsharaf24@gmail.com (J.M.S.); peter.henderson@mountsinai.org (P.W.H.)
[2] SUNY Downstate Medical School, SUNY Downstate Health Sciences University, Brooklyn, NY 11203, USA; christopher.alessandro@downstate.edu
[3] The American Medical Program, Tel Aviv University, Tel Aviv 6997801, Israel; rabinovich1@mail.tau.ac.il
* Correspondence: alice.yao@mountsinai.org; Tel.: +1-212-241-4410

Abstract: The expansion of robotic surgery has led to developments in robotic-assisted breast reconstruction techniques. Specifically, robotic flap harvest is being evaluated to help maximize operative reliability and reduce donor site morbidity without compromising flap success. Many publications are feasibility studies or technical descriptions; few cohort analyses exist. This systematic review aims to characterize trends in robotic autologous breast reconstruction and provide a summative analysis of their results. A systematic review was conducted using PubMed, Medline, Scopus, and Web of Science to evaluate robot use in breast reconstruction. Studies dated from 2006 to 2022 were identified and analyzed using the Preferred Reporting Items for Systematic Reviews and Meta-Analyses (PRISMA) guidelines. Full-text, peer-reviewed, English-language, and human subject studies were included. Non-breast reconstruction articles, commentary, expert opinion, editor's letter, and duplicate studies were excluded. A total of 17 full-text articles were analyzed. The two robotic breast procedures identified were the deep inferior epigastric perforator (DIEP) and the latissimus dorsi (LD) flap. Results showed comparable complication rates and increased operative times compared to NSQIP data on their corresponding open techniques. Additional findings reported in studies included patient reported outcomes, incision lengths, and downward trends in operative time with consecutive procedures. The available data in the literature confirms that robotic surgery is a promising alternative to traditional open methods of breast reconstruction following mastectomy.

Keywords: robotic surgery; autologous breast reconstruction; surgical innovation; robotic-assisted surgery; robotic breast surgery; robotic plastic surgery

1. Introduction

Robotic surgery has emerged over the past two decades as an exciting new tool in the surgical armamentarium. Surgical robots have gained traction in numerous fields, including general surgery, orthopedics, gynecology, urology, otolaryngology, and plastic surgery [1–6]. The da Vinci® robot was first cleared by the United States Food and Drug Administration (FDA) in 2001 for use in laparoscopic surgical procedures such as removal of the gallbladder and surgery for severe heartburn [7]. Robotic surgery has shown immense promise in reducing adverse outcomes; for example, nerve sparing robotic-assisted prostatectomy has been shown to preserve continence and sexual function [8]. More recently, robotic surgery has been introduced into breast reconstruction, with promising operative and postoperative outcomes.

Despite its growing use, literature on robotic autologous breast reconstruction is limited and heterogeneous. As a newer technology, it is imperative that outcomes and associated costs are critically evaluated. Understanding the intra- and postoperative advantages and disadvantages of robotic breast surgery can better aid surgeons in planning and facilitating breast surgical care and in understanding indications for use of robotics in breast surgery. As technological innovations continue to allow improved operative procedures, it is crucial to assess the advantages and pitfalls of new surgical techniques integrated with technology. Thus, the aim of this systematic review is to characterize the current trends in robotic autologous breast reconstruction (RABR) and provide insight on the current advantages and areas for improvement for each flap described in the literature.

2. Materials and Methods

2.1. Study Design

A systematic review was conducted using the PubMed, Medline, Scopus, and Web of Science databases to identify RABR articles from January 2006–February 2022, in accordance with the Preferred Reporting Items for Systematic Reviews and Meta-Analyses (PRISMA) guidelines (Figure 1). This systematic review has been registered with PROSPERO (CRD42023425313). Boolean operators were used to identify articles on "Robotic breast surgery", "Robotic breast reconstruction", AND "outcome" OR "trend" OR "satisfaction". Additional searches were performed to identify common RABR procedures, namely "robotic deep inferior epigastric perforator" and "robotic latissimus dorsi flap". The searches were carried out using the full procedure name, as well as their common abbreviations ("robotic DIEP" and "robotic LD"). No restrictions were used.

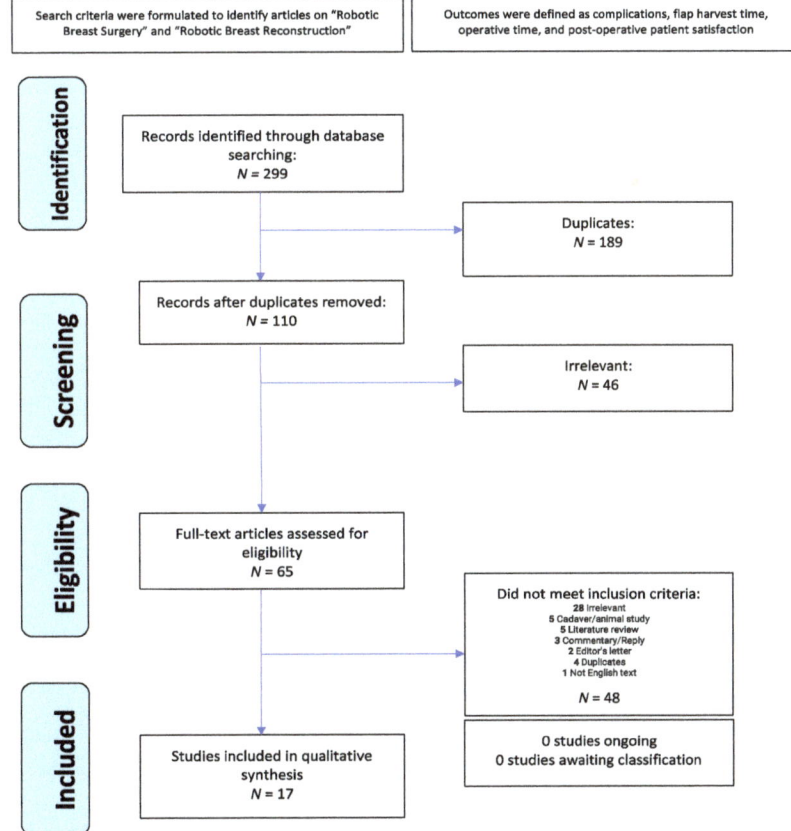

Figure 1. Preferred reporting items for systematic reviews and meta-analyses (PRISMA) protocol.

Articles were included if the following criteria were met: the full-text article was available, the article was peer-reviewed, all text was written in English, and all subjects were humans who underwent RABR following any type of mastectomy. Non-breast reconstruction-related articles, non-autologous breast reconstruction studies, cadaveric/non-human subject studies, commentary/expert opinion/editor's letter, review articles, and duplicate studies were excluded.

2.2. Data Collection

Two independent reviewers (A.A. and D.R.) screened titles and abstracts for inclusion. Next, four independent reviewers (N.R., T.I., A.A., and D.R.) extracted the following data from the full-text articles: study title, author, year of publication, country of publication, journal of publication, sample size, study aim, patient age, type of robot used, type of flap, immediate vs. delayed reconstruction, reconstruction stage, robotic technique, total operative time, robotic time, and complications (Table 1). Two independent reviewers (A.Y. and P.H.) resolved any conflicts among reviewers.

2.3. Data Analysis

The total mean operating time for RABR was calculated by weighing each full-text article by its sample size. Study times were also stratified by immediate or delayed operation types. DIEP and LD procedure times were subsequently compared to flap procedures reported in the National Surgical Quality Improvement Program (NSQIP) database, a nationally validated, risk-adjusted database tracking surgical outcomes [9]. This database acted as the control group and was specifically filtered for DIEP flap breast reconstruction via Current Procedural Terminology (CPT) code 19364 and LD flap reconstruction via CPT code 19361.

Complications from each full-text article were also mapped to relevant NSQIP database complications and to ICD-9 or ICD-10 code sets. Pearson's chi-square or Fisher exact tests were used to determine associations between surgery type and complications, and odds ratios were then calculated to compare these complication rates.

Statistical analysis was performed by author C.A. using SPSS Statistics for Windows, version 28 (SPSS Inc., Chicago, IL, USA).

2.4. Outcomes

The primary outcome of interest was the presence of postoperative complications. Secondary outcomes included operative time, robotic-assisted flap harvest time, robotic technique, and number of reconstruction stages.

Table 1. Summary of extracted data across all studies.

Latissimus Dorsi

Authors (Year)	Country	Study Design	Sample Size	Patient Age (Mean ± SD)	Type of Robot	Immediate or Delayed Reconstruction	Laterality	Number of Reconstruction Stages	Robotic Technique	Mean Total Operative Time (Minutes)	Mean Robotic Time (Minutes)	Complications
Chung et al. (2015) [10]	South Korea	Retrospective case series	12	35.8 ± 11.8	da Vinci S *	Immediate (n = 4) Delayed (n = 8)	Unilateral	One-stage (n = 4) Two-stage (n = 3) Not applicable (n = 5) **	MP	400.4	85.8	Contour irregularity: 8% (n = 1)
Clemens, M. W., Kronowitz, S., Selber, J. C. (2014) [11]	USA	Retrospective cohort study	12	54.3	da Vinci *	Delayed-Immediate	Unilateral	Two-stage	MP	92	Not specified	Infection: 8% (n = 1) Unplanned OR: 8.3% (n = 1)
Houvenaeghel et al. (2020) [12]	France	Retrospective cohort study	35	51.2 ± 13.5	da Vinci Si: (n = 12) da Vinci Xi: (n = 23) *	Immediate NSM	Unilateral	One-stage	MP-Breast	337	Not specified	Dorsal seroma: 25.7% (n = 9) Hemorrhage/Reoperation: 2.9% (n = 1)
Houvenaeghel et al. (2020) [13]	France	Retrospective comparative study	46	58.1 ± 14.2	da Vinci Si (n = 17) da Vinci Xi (n = 23) *	Immediate SSM	Unilateral	One-stage	MP-Breast	290.5	Not specified	Dorsal seroma: 26% (n = 12) Dorsal bleeding: 2% (n = 1) Infection: 4% (n = 2) Reoperation: 4% (n = 2)
Joo et al. (2021) [14]	South Korea	Case report	1	40	da Vinci SP *	Immediate	Unilateral	One-stage	SP	328	115	None
Lai et al. (2018) [15]	Taiwan	Case report	2	47 ± 0.5	da Vinci Si *	Immediate	Unilateral	One-stage	MP	263	178.5	Seroma: 100% (n = 2)
Moon et al. (2020) [16]	South Korea	Retrospective cohort study	21	29.9 ± 6.8	da Vinci Xi *	Immediate	Unilateral	One-stage	MP-Scapula	295	143	Seroma: 19% (n = 4) Axillary wound complication: 5% (n = 1)
Selber, J. C., Baumann, D. P., Holsinger, C. F. (2012) [17]	USA	Case report	6	Not specified	da Vinci S *	Immediate (n = 3) Delayed (n = 3)	Unilateral	Two-stage	MP	Not specified	111	Transient nerve palsy: 16% (n = 1)
Winocour et al. (2020) [18]	USA	Retrospective review	25	51 ± 9.7	da Vinci *	Not specified	Unilateral	Not specified	MP	366	Not specified	Seroma: 16% (n = 4)

Table 1. *Cont.*

Deep Inferior Epigastric Perforator

Authors (Year)	Country	Study Design	Sample Size	Patient Age (Mean ± SD)	Type of Robot	Immediate or Delayed Reconstruction	Laterality	Number of Reconstruction Stages	Robotic Technique	Mean Total Operative Time (Minutes)	Mean Robotic Time (Minutes)	Complications
Bishop et al. (2022) [19]	USA	Retrospective case series	21	54.6 ± 7.6	Not specified	Not specified	Unilateral	Not specified	TAPP	425.3	44.8	Surgical site occurrence (n = 5) Delayed wound healing (n = 1)
Choi et al. (2021) [20]	South Korea	Retrospective case series	17	Not specified	da Vinci SP *	Not specified	Not specified	Not specified	TEP (using single port)	487	65	Not specified
Daar et al. (2022) [21]	USA	Retrospective case series	4	52 ± 6.9	da Vinci Xi *	Both	Bilateral (n = 3) Unilateral (n = 1)	Both	TAPP	717.6	Not specified	Wound dehiscence: 50% (n = 2)
Gundlapalli et al. (2018) [22]	USA	Case report	1	51	da Vinci *	Delayed	Unilateral	Two-stage	TAPP	471	60	None
Kurlander et al. (2021) [23]	USA	Case series	13	50 ± 9.9	Not specified	Immediate	Not specified	One-stage	TAPP	Not specified	Not specified	None
Lee et al. (2022) [24]	South Korea	Retrospective cohort study	21	48.5 ± 6.6	da Vinci SP *	Immediate	Unilateral	One-stage	TAPP	509	Not specified	Flap loss (n = 1), Fat necrosis (n = 2)
Piper et al. (2021) [25]	USA	Case report	4	50.25 ± 8.2	da Vinci Xi *	Immediate	Not specified	One-stage	TAPP	Not specified	45	None
Shakir et al. (2021) [26]	USA	Retrospective cohort study	3	53.2 ± 8.5	da Vinci Xi *	Delayed	Unilateral	Two-stage	TAPP	535	40	None

Addendum: * = Intuitive Surgical, Sunnyvale, CA; ** = Poland Syndrome; MP: Multi-port; NSM: Nipple-sparing mastectomy; SP: Single-port; SSM: Skin-sparing mastectomy; TAPP: Transabdominal pre-peritoneal; TEP: Total extraperitoneal.

3. Results

Of the 299 identified articles, a total of 17 full-text articles published from 2006–2022 met inclusion criteria. There were 5 retrospective cohort studies, 5 case reports, 4 retrospective case series, 1 case series, 1 retrospective review, and 1 retrospective comparative study. The mean age of patients was 48.4 years. A total of 84 patients underwent deep inferior epigastric perforator (DIEP) flap breast reconstruction, and 160 patients underwent latissimus dorsi (LD) flap breast reconstruction. The most common type of reconstruction performed was an immediate, one-stage reconstruction. The da Vinci Si robot was the most commonly used device. Other devices used were the da Vinci SP, the da Vinci S, and the da Vinci Xi (Table 1). For all robotic procedures studied, mean total operative time was 394 min and mean robotic time was 88 min. RABR was negatively associated with the need to return to the operating room (OR = 0.149) compared to NSQIP data (Figure 2).

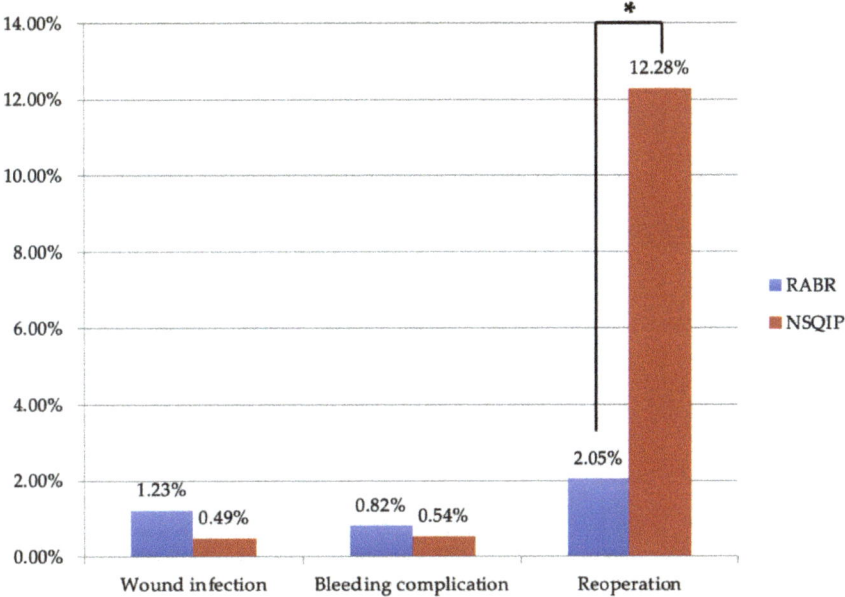

Figure 2. Comparison between RABR and NSQIP complication profiles. Key: RABR: Robotic Autologous Breast Reconstruction; NSQIP: National Surgical Quality Improvement Program. *—indicates significance, $p < 0.05$.

3.1. Latissimus Dorsi

Operative techniques used for breast reconstruction with LD were multi-port (MP), MP with breast port access (MP-Breast), MP with scapular port access (MP-Scapula), and single-port (SP) (Figure 3). For patients undergoing LD flap reconstruction, 42 complications were reported (Table 2). Complications ranged from bleeding to seroma formation and nerve palsy. One patient experienced contour irregularity following an LD flap reconstruction. The most common complication among LD flaps was dorsal donor site seroma formation. On average, SP robotic operative time was shortest longest in comparison to other operative techniques, though there was only one case demonstrated (Table 3). Total operative time for LD robotic-assisted procedures was longer (296 min) than NSQIP reported data (256 min) (Figure 4).

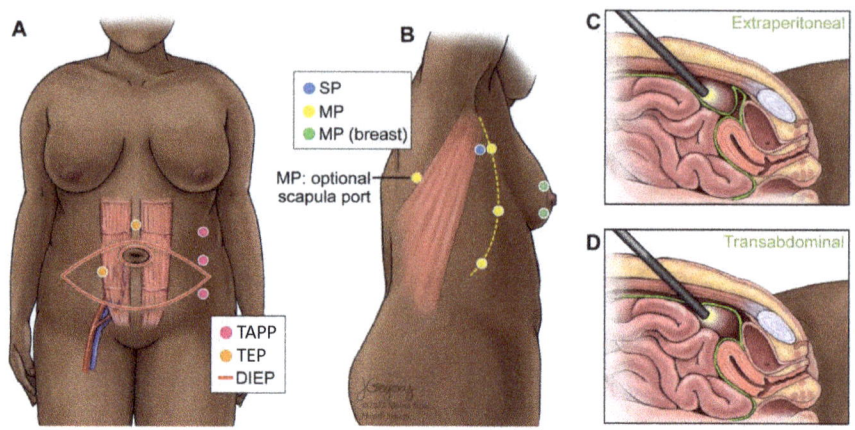

Figure 3. Schematic of port access sites for latissimus dorsi and DIEP flap robotic-assisted surgery. (**A**) Port site variations for the robotic DIEP. (**B**) Port site variations for the robotic LD. (**C**) Depth of port for DIEP-TEP. (**D**) Depth of port for DIEP-TAPP. Key: DIEP: Deep inferior epigastric perforator; MP: Multi-port; SP: Single-port; TAPP: Transabdominal pre-peritoneal; TEP: Total extraperitoneal.

Table 2. Complications by flap type.

Type of Flap	Complication	Number of Patients (n)	Percentage (%)
Latissimus Dorsi			
LD (n = 160)	Donor site seroma	31	19.3%
	Re-operation	3	1.8%
	Contour irregularity	1	<1%
	Infection	3	1.8%
	Hemorrhage requiring reoperation	1	<1%
	Dorsal bleeding	1	<1%
	Other wound complication (axillary)	1	<1%
	Nerve palsy	1	<1%
	Total	42	19%
Deep Inferior Epigastric Perforator			
Type of Flap	Complication	Number of Patients (n)	Percentage (%)
DIEP (n = 84)	Wound dehiscence	3	3.6%
	Flap loss	1	1.2%
	Fat necrosis	2	2.4%
	Other (not specified)	4	4.8%
	Total	10	12%

Key: DIEP: Deep inferior epigastric perforator; LD: Latissimus dorsi.

Table 3. Patient distribution and mean operative time by surgical approach.

Mean Operative Time: Latissimus Dorsi				
Robotic Technique	Number of Procedures	Mean Operative Time (minutes)		Ratio Robotic to Total Operative Time
		Total	Robotic	
MP	57	280	125	44%
MP-Breast	81	314	—	—
MP-Scapula	21	295	143	48%
SP	1	328	115	35%

Table 3. *Cont.*

	Mean Operative Time: Deep Inferior Epigastric Perforator			Ratio Robotic to Total Operative Time
Robotic Technique	**Number of Procedures**	**Mean Operative Time (minutes)**		
		Total	Robotic	
TAPP	67	531	47	8%
TEP	17	487	65	13%

Key: MP: Multi-port; SP: Single-port; TAPP: Transabdominal pre-peritoneal; TEP: Total extraperitoneal.

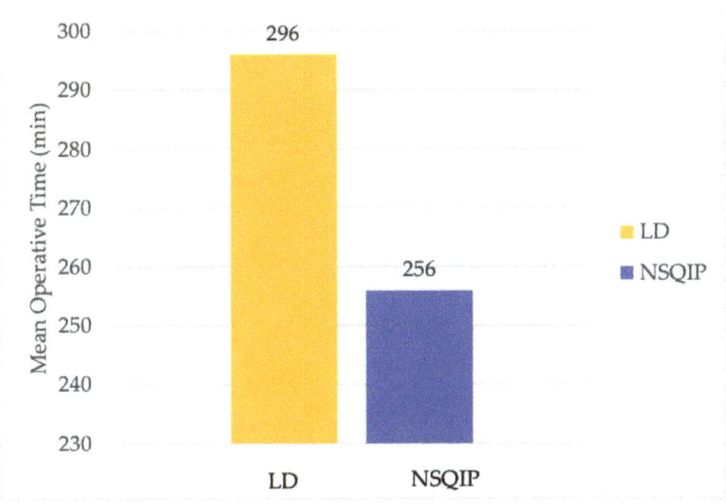

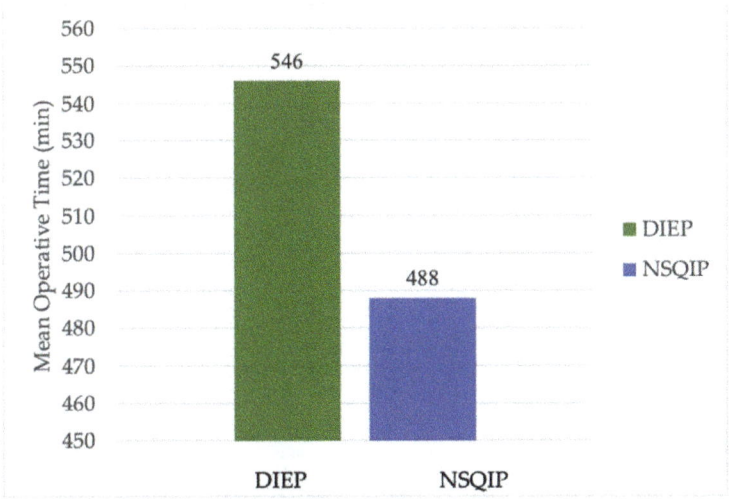

Figure 4. Mean operative times by reconstruction type. Key: DIEP: Deep inferior epigastric perforator; LD: Latissimus dorsi; NSQIP: National Surgical Quality Improvement Program.

3.2. Deep Inferior Epigastric Perforator

Operative techniques for the DIEP were transabdominal pre-peritoneal (TAPP) vs. total extraperitoneal (TEP) approaches for the DIEP (Figure 3). The TAPP procedures were performed with a multi-port device. The TEP procedure was completed with a single-port (da Vinci SP). For patients undergoing DIEP flap reconstruction, 10 complications were reported (Table 2). The most common specified complication among DIEP flaps was wound dehiscence (Table 2). On average, TAPP robotic operative time was shorter in comparison to TEP (Table 3). Total operative time for DIEP robotic-assisted procedures was longer (546 min) than NSQIP reported data (488 min) (Figure 4).

4. Discussion

Breast reconstruction rates continue to rise, highlighting the importance of diverse treatment options and favorable outcomes. Numerous factors, such as age, socioeconomic status, geographic location, ethnicity, and patient preference, influence the decision to undergo breast reconstruction following mastectomy [27]. Reconstruction has been linked to lower anxiety and depression levels and improved quality of life compared to mastectomy alone [28,29].

In recent years, robotic mastectomy has emerged as an innovative technique in breast cancer surgery, offering potential advantages such as reduced blood loss, smaller incisions, faster recovery times, and improved cosmetic outcomes [30]. As the adoption of robotic mastectomy increases, RABR may serve to further enhance patient outcomes and satisfaction.

Robotic reconstruction, which offers potential advantages such as tremor elimination, increased surgical dexterity, and minimally invasive approaches, is a promising technique to address the ever-present demand for improved reconstructive outcomes. Further research and technological advancements may help to make robotic reconstruction more accessible and appealing, ultimately decreasing operative morbidity and improving patients' psychological well-being and quality of life after mastectomy.

Comparing operative times, complication rates, patient-reported outcome measures (PROMs), and fascial incision data from robotic and traditional reconstructive surgery literature can provide valuable insights into the feasibility of robotic reconstruction techniques.

4.1. Operative Time

It is not surprising that robotic procedures take longer compared to their open counterparts due to the need for device setup and troubleshooting. In a comparison of operative times for deep inferior epigastric perforator (DIEP) flap breast reconstruction, robotic-assisted procedures averaged 546 min, while data from the National Surgical Quality Improvement Program (NSQIP) reported an average of 488 min for non-robotic procedures. Issa et al. found mean operative times of 506.3 min for immediate bilateral DIEP flap reconstruction using an open approach and 464.8 min for delayed bilateral DIEP flap reconstruction [31]. Similarly, the robotic LD averaged a longer operative time than open (296 and 256 min, respectively). Despite the slightly longer duration for robotic-assisted procedures, the difference in operative time remains relatively modest when compared to non-robotic methods. While the robotic method certainly requires more training and longer operative time initially as an investment, increased experience with robotic surgery may lead to improved operative times and efficiency, as suggested by Moon et al., who reported a downward trend in operative times with each subsequent case performed [32].

4.2. Complication Rates

Complication rates between RABR and traditional techniques appear to be comparable, as shown in Figure 2. Due to the nature of our study, direct comparison with NSQIP data is limited; however, existing literature supports similar findings. Clemens et al. reported a 16.7% overall complication rate for robotic assisted LD versus 37.5% for traditional open latissimus dorsi (LD) reconstruction [11], while Houvenaeghel et al. found rates of 28.6%

for robotic assisted LD compared to 51.4% for the traditional LD approach [12]. Notably, Bishop et al. observed decreased pain on the robotic side for patients who underwent bilateral DIEP surgery with one robotic and one open procedure [19]. While the robotic re-operation rate in our study was promising and proved to be statistically lower than the NSQIP data, the robotic procedures are new and the follow-up time is relatively short, so may not account for re-operation events further in the future.

4.3. Patient-Reported Outcome Measures

Several studies have investigated patient-reported outcome measures (PROMs) for robotic-assisted breast reconstruction (RABR). Chung et al. found high mean satisfaction scores across various categories, such as general satisfaction, scar formation, and breast aesthetics [10]. Joo et al. used the BREAST-Q tool and reported higher mean overall scores for RABR patients compared to those who underwent traditional breast reconstruction [14]. Similarly, Moon et al. observed favorable mean PROMs for improvement in chest deformity, chest symmetry, scar formation, and overall satisfaction [16]. These findings suggest that RABR is associated with positive patient-reported outcomes; however, a prospective study directly comparing BREAST-Q outcomes of robotic and traditional techniques has not been conducted.

4.4. Incision Length

The minimally invasive nature of robotic surgery results in shorter scars in latissimus-based breast reconstruction [14] and limited fascial incisions in abdominally based breast reconstruction. Several studies have reported fascial incision lengths for DIEP flaps, highlighting the potential benefits of a smaller incision. While long-term data is limited, a reduced fascial incision length may decrease the risks of hernia and bulge, which are common and potentially underreported complications of DIEP flaps. Reported robotic fascial incision lengths ranged from 1.5 cm to 7 cm. Kurlander et al. discussed using preoperative computed tomography angiography (CTA) to determine robotic DIEP candidacy and reported a mean fascial incision length of 3.5 cm in their preselected population. This is markedly shorter than the mean fascial length of a traditional open DIEP flap of 13.3 cm [33]. Given the potential postoperative benefits of reduced long-term risk for abdominal bulge or hernia, plastic surgeons should consider this metric when evaluating the robotic approach.

Although robotic-assisted breast reconstruction has many apparent benefits, potential drawbacks of robotic-assisted surgery must also be considered. These include longer operative times, variable postoperative outcomes, and increased financial burden [34–36]. The time-consuming start-up, docking, and setup of the robot, as well as its occupation of operating room space, may impact operative efficiency. The choice between a single-port or multi-port robotic system can also affect the docking process, camera flexibility, and potential for robotic arm collisions [14]. The controversy surrounding robotic surgery stems from its challenge to the status quo of reconstructive procedures and the financial and technical obstacles it presents. More research is needed to form definitive conclusions, such as the number of procedures required to optimize operative time when using a robotic approach, the optimal device and technique to use for each procedure, and the relative risk/benefit ratio of outcomes such as bleeding and hernia.

To our knowledge, this represents the first systematic review that compares complication types and rates for robotic-assisted breast reconstruction (RABR) with nationally collected data on surgical outcomes in traditional open flap autologous breast reconstruction. We further characterized RABR by surgical technique and compared operative times among procedures. Previous systematic reviews have also assessed robotic techniques in autologous breast reconstruction. Donnelly et al. conducted a systematic review with findings comparable to ours, focusing on financial cost and the total length of the hospital stay as key outcomes [37]. Our study builds upon their work by incorporating data from Medline, PubMed, and Web of Science to capture a larger pool of published studies.

Dobbs et al. conducted a comprehensive, systematic review in 2017, revealing a steady increase in publications on robotic surgery in general over the past 20 years, from 168 in 2000 to over 2000 in 2014 [6]. There seems to be a similarly growing interest in robotic surgery among plastic surgeons in publications and conferences, emphasizing the need for further evaluation and in-depth study of its benefits and drawbacks.

This study rigorously characterizes the role of robotic surgery in autologous breast reconstruction, from its first published article in 2004 to the present day. However, it has limitations and challenges. Primarily, our findings are based on case reports, case series, and non-randomized cohort studies, which may contain biases. Consequently, conclusions should be approached with caution.

Over half of the included studies did not differentiate between total operative and robotic time, making it difficult to determine if the robotic component influences operative time or financial costs. Furthermore, studies lacked consistent reporting of patient demographics and comorbidities, which are crucial factors in postoperative complications. This makes it challenging to ascertain if robotic surgeries or specific flap types lead to a higher incidence of complications compared to traditional techniques.

Direct comparison with NSQIP data also has its limitations, as the CPT code for breast reconstruction with free flap (19364) does not distinguish between abdominal donor site (DIEP) versus other types of flaps such as thigh or gluteal. However, we expect the data to trend toward abdominal flaps as they are much more commonly performed than other flaps for breast reconstruction [38]. The NSQIP database also does not specify between unilateral and bilateral DIEP flap reconstruction. As such, we were unable to draw a direct comparison between unilateral and bilateral operative times for NSQIP-reported data and the data obtained from this systematic review. Lastly, as robotic technology is still emerging in plastic surgery, these preliminary results may not fully represent the potential of RABR.

As the field of RABR is still developing, future studies should focus on conducting prospective cohort studies in eligible patients to compare the efficacy of robotic and traditional surgical techniques across various free and pedicled flaps. Additionally, it is crucial for studies to emphasize the significance of patient selection when reporting results, allowing for a better understanding of the ideal candidates for RABR and facilitating more tailored approaches in breast reconstruction.

The widely used robotic systems in surgical procedures, including the RABR procedures included in this analysis, were not designed with reconstructive surgery in mind. Although the system has demonstrated potential benefits, it is crucial to acknowledge its limitations in the context of breast reconstruction. These limitations include high costs, a steep learning curve, ergonomic considerations, limited haptic feedback, bulky equipment, and a lack of dedicated instruments tailored for plastic surgery [39]. Despite these challenges, advancements in technology hold promise for the development of future robotic systems that can overcome these limitations. Improved haptic feedback, miniaturization, dedicated instruments, cost reduction, and integration with imaging technologies may enhance the effectiveness and versatility of robotic assistance in plastic surgery. The Symani Surgical System® (Medical Microinstruments, MMI, Calci, Italy) is a relatively novel robotic microsurgical system that consists of enhanced magnification and flexible robotic arms that can reach into deeper anatomical regions [40]. It has been utilized for numerous plastic surgery procedures, including lymphedema and autologous breast reconstruction via the profunda artery perforator flap [40]. Surgeons continue to engage with new robotic surgical systems in reconstructive surgery and microsurgery, contributing to innovation and advancement in the field of plastic surgery.

5. Conclusions

Operative efficiency, postoperative clinical outcomes, and patient satisfaction are all of great importance to the plastic surgeon. Robotic-assisted breast reconstruction has been shown to be a feasible procedure with advantages including smaller skin or fascial incision sizes and reduced complication rates. Smaller fascial incision sizes may lead to decreased long-term postoperative complications, such as abdominal hernia and chronic postoperative pain, though these complications can take many years to present. There is still limited data in this field regarding operative efficiency, cost, and maximal patient benefit. A continued effort to understand how robotic assistance can aid the plastic surgeon will hopefully shed more light on the robot as a tool of the future for breast reconstruction.

Author Contributions: Conceptualization, P.W.H.; methodology, N.R., D.R., A.A.A. and T.J.I.; formal analysis, C.J.A.; investigation, N.R.; resources, N.R.; data curation, N.R.; writing—original draft preparation, N.R. and J.M.S.; writing—review and editing, A.A.A., T.J.I., P.W.H. and A.Y.; visualization, N.R.; supervision, P.W.H. and A.Y.; project administration, P.W.H. and A.Y. All authors have read and agreed to the published version of the manuscript.

Funding: This research received no external funding.

Institutional Review Board Statement: Not applicable.

Informed Consent Statement: Not applicable.

Data Availability Statement: No new data were created or analyzed in this study. Data sharing is not applicable to this article. No review protocol was prepared for this study.

Acknowledgments: The authors would like to acknowledge Jill Gregory at the Icahn School of Medicine at Mount Sinai for her illustrative contributions.

Conflicts of Interest: The authors declare no conflict of interest.

References

1. Deutsch, G.B.; Sathyanarayana, S.A.; Gunabushanam, V.; Mishra, N.; Rubach, E.; Zemon, H.; Klein, J.D.S.; DeNoto, G. Robotic vs. laparoscopic colorectal surgery: An institutional experience. *Surg. Endosc.* **2012**, *26*, 956–963. [CrossRef] [PubMed]
2. Gala, R.B.; Margulies, R.; Steinberg, A.; Murphy, M.; Lukban, J.; Jeppson, P.; Aschkenazi, S.; Olivera, C.; South, M.; Lowenstein, L.; et al. Systematic Review of Robotic Surgery in Gynecology: Robotic Techniques Compared With Laparoscopy and Laparotomy. *J. Minim. Invasive Gynecol.* **2014**, *21*, 353–361. [CrossRef] [PubMed]
3. Li, C.; Wang, L.; Perka, C.; Trampuz, A. Clinical application of robotic orthopedic surgery: A bibliometric study. *BMC Musculoskelet. Disord.* **2021**, *22*, 968. [CrossRef] [PubMed]
4. Honda, M.; Morizane, S.; Hikita, K.; Takenaka, A. Current status of robotic surgery in urology. *Asian J. Endosc. Surg.* **2017**, *11*, 372–381. [CrossRef] [PubMed]
5. Maan, Z.N.; Gibbins, N.; Al-Jabri, T.; D'Souza, A.R. The use of robotics in otolaryngology-head and neck surgery: A systematic review. *Am. J. Otolaryngol.* **2012**, *33*, 137–146. [CrossRef]
6. Dobbs, T.D.; Cundy, O.; Samarendra, H.; Khan, K.; Whitaker, I.S. A Systematic Review of the Role of Robotics in Plastic and Reconstructive Surgery-From Inception to the Future. *Front. Surg.* **2017**, *4*, 66. [CrossRef]
7. Meadows, M. Robots lend a helping hand to surgeons. *FDA Consum.* **2002**, *36*, 10–15.
8. Tewari, A.K.; Ali, A.; Metgud, S.; Theckumparampil, N.; Srivastava, A.; Khani, F.; Robinson, B.D.; Gumpeni, N.; Shevchuk, M.M.; Durand, M.; et al. Functional outcomes following robotic prostatectomy using a thermal, traction free risk-stratified grades of nerve sparing. *World J. Urol.* **2013**, *31*, 471–480. [CrossRef]
9. Raval, M.V.; Pawlik, T.M. Practical Guide to Surgical Data Sets: National Surgical Quality Improvement Program (NSQIP) and Pediatric NSQIP. In *JAMA Guide to Statistics and Methods*; Livingston, E.H., Lewis, R.J., Eds.; McGraw Hill: New York, NY, USA, 2019.
10. Chung, J.H.; You, H.J.; Kim, H.S.; Lee, B.-I.; Park, S.-H.; Yoon, E.-S. A novel technique for robot assisted latissimus dorsi flap harvest. *J. Plast. Reconstr. Aesthet. Surg.* **2015**, *68*, 966–972. [CrossRef]
11. Clemens, M.W.; Kronowitz, S.; Selber, J.C. Robotic-assisted latissimus dorsi harvest in delayed-immediate breast reconstruction. *Semin. Plast. Surg.* **2014**, *28*, 20–25. [CrossRef]
12. Houvenaeghel, G.; Cohen, M.; Ribeiro, S.R.; Barrou, J.; Heinemann, M.; Frayret, C.; Lambaudie, E.; Bannier, M. Robotic Nipple-Sparing Mastectomy and Immediate Breast Reconstruction With Robotic Latissimus Dorsi Flap Harvest: Technique and Results. *Surg. Innov.* **2020**, *27*, 481–491. [CrossRef]
13. Houvenaeghel, G.; El Hajj, H.; Schmitt, A.; Cohen, M.; Rua, S.; Barrou, J.; Lambaudie, E.; Bannier, M. Robotic-assisted skin sparing mastectomy and immediate reconstruction using latissimus dorsi flap a new effective and safe technique: A comparative study. *Surg. Oncol.* **2020**, *35*, 406–411. [CrossRef]
14. Joo, O.Y.; Song, S.Y.; Lew, D.H.; Park, H.S.; Lee, D.W. Robotic harvest of a latissimus dorsi flap using a single-port surgical robotic system in breast reconstruction. *Arch. Plast. Surg.* **2021**, *48*, 577–582. [CrossRef]

15. Lai, H.W.; Chen, S.T.; Lin, S.L.; Lin, Y.L.; Wu, H.K.; Pai, S.H.; Chen, D.R.; Kuo, S.J. Technique for single axillary incision robotic assisted quadrantectomy and immediate partial breast reconstruction with robotic latissimus dorsi flap harvest for breast cancer: A case report. *Medicine* **2018**, *97*, e11373. [CrossRef] [PubMed]
16. Moon, K.C.; Yeo, H.D.; Yoon, E.S.; Lee, B.; Park, S.; Chung, J.; Lee, H. Robotic-assisted latissimus dorsi muscle flap for autologous chest reconstruction in poland syndrome. *J. Plast. Reconstr. Aesthet. Surg.* **2020**, *73*, 1506–1513. [CrossRef] [PubMed]
17. Selber, J.C.; Baumann, D.P.; Holsinger, C.F. Robotic harvest of the latissimus dorsi muscle: Laboratory and clinical experience. *J. Reconstr. Microsurg.* **2012**, *28*, 457–464. [CrossRef]
18. Winocour, S.; Tarassoli, S.; Chu, C.K.; Liu, J.; Clemens, M.W.; Selber, J.C. Comparing Outcomes of Robotically Assisted Latissimus Dorsi Harvest to the Traditional Open Approach in Breast Reconstruction. *Plast. Reconstr. Surg.* **2020**, *146*, 1221–1225. [CrossRef] [PubMed]
19. Bishop, S.N.; Asaad, M.; Liu, J.; Chu, C.K.M.; Clemens, M.W.M.; Kapur, S.S.M.; Largo, R.D.M.; Selber, J.C.M. Robotic Harvest of the Deep Inferior Epigastric Perforator Flap for Breast Reconstruction: A Case Series. *Plast. Reconstr. Surg.* **2022**, *149*, 1073–1077. [CrossRef]
20. Choi, J.H.; Song, S.Y.; Park, H.S.; Kim, C.H.; Kim, J.Y.; Lew, D.H.; Roh, T.S.; Lee, D.W. Robotic DIEP Flap Harvest through a Totally Extraperitoneal Approach Using a Single-Port Surgical Robotic System. *Plast. Reconstr. Surg.* **2021**, *148*, 304–307. [CrossRef] [PubMed]
21. Daar, D.A.; Anzai, L.M.; Vranis, N.M.; Schulster, M.L.; Frey, J.D.; Jun, M.; Zhao, L.C.; Levine, J.P. Robotic deep inferior epigastric perforator flap harvest in breast reconstruction. *Microsurgery* **2022**, *42*, 319–325. [CrossRef]
22. Gundlapalli, V.S.; Ogunleye, A.A.; Scott, K.; Wenzinger, E.; Ulm, J.P.; Tavana, L.; Pullatt, R.C.; Delaney, K.O. Robotic-assisted deep inferior epigastric artery perforator flap abdominal harvest for breast reconstruction: A case report. *Microsurgery* **2018**, *38*, 702–705. [CrossRef] [PubMed]
23. Kurlander, D.E.; Le-Petross, H.T.; Shuck, J.W.; Butler, C.E.; Selber, J.C. Robotic DIEP Patient Selection: Analysis of CT Angiography. *Plast. Reconstr. Surg. Glob. Open.* **2021**, *9*, e3970. [CrossRef] [PubMed]
24. Lee, M.J.; Won, J.; Song, S.Y.; Park, H.S.; Kim, J.Y.; Shin, H.J.; Kwon, Y.I.; Lee, D.W.; Kim, N.Y. Clinical outcomes following robotic versus conventional DIEP flap in breast reconstruction: A retrospective matched study. *Front. Oncol.* **2022**, *12*, 989231. [CrossRef]
25. Piper, M.; Ligh, C.A.; Shakir, S.; Messa, C.; Soriano, I.; Kanchwala, S. Minimally invasive robotic-assisted harvest of the deep inferior epigastric perforator flap for autologous breast reconstruction. *J. Plast. Reconstr. Aesthet. Surg.* **2021**, *74*, 890–930. [CrossRef]
26. Shakir, S.; Spencer, A.B.; Piper, M.; Kozak, G.M.; Soriano, I.S.; Kanchwala, S.K. Laparoscopy allows the harvest of the DIEP flap with shorter fascial incisions as compared to endoscopic harvest: A single surgeon retrospective cohort study. *J. Plast. Reconstr. Aesthetic Surg.* **2021**, *74*, 1203–1212. [CrossRef]
27. Morrow, M.; Scott, S.K.; Menck, H.R.; Mustoe, T.A.; Winchester, D.P. Factors influencing the use of breast reconstruction postmastectomy: A National Cancer Database study. *J. Am. Coll. Surg.* **2001**, *192*, 1–8. [CrossRef]
28. Morrow, M.; Li, Y.; Alderman, A.K.; Jagsi, R.; Hamilton, A.S.; Graff, J.J.; Hawley, S.T.; Katz, S.J. Access to breast reconstruction after mastectomy and patient perspectives on reconstruction decision making. *JAMA Surg.* **2014**, *149*, 1015–1021. [CrossRef] [PubMed]
29. Bishop, S.N.; Selber, J.C. Minimally invasive robotic breast reconstruction surgery. *Gland. Surg.* **2021**, *10*, 469–478. [CrossRef]
30. Houvenaeghel, G.; Barrou, J.; Jauffret, C.; Rua, S.; Sabiani, L.; Van Troy, A.; Buttarelli, M.; Blache, G.; Lambaudie, E.; Cohen, M.; et al. Robotic Versus Conventional Nipple-Sparing Mastectomy with Immediate Breast Reconstruction. *Front. Oncol.* **2021**, *11*, 637049. [CrossRef]
31. Issa, C.J.; Lu, S.M.; Boudiab, E.M.; DeSano, J.D.; Sachanandani, N.S.; Powers, J.M.; Chaiyasate, K. Comparing Plastic Surgeon Operative Time for DIEP Flap Breast Reconstruction: 2-stage More Efficient than 1-stage? *Plast. Reconstr. Surg. Glob. Open* **2021**, *9*, e3608. [CrossRef]
32. Moon, J.; Lee, J.; Lee, D.W.; Lee, H.S.; Nam, D.J.; Kim, M.J.; Kim, N.Y.; Park, H.S. Postoperative pain assessment of robotic nipple-sparing mastectomy with immediate prepectoral prosthesis breast reconstruction: A comparison with conventional nipple-sparing mastectomy. *Int. J. Med. Sci.* **2021**, *18*, 2409–2416. [CrossRef]
33. Bailey, E.; Chen, B.; Nelson, W.; Nosik, S.; Fortunato, R.; Moreira, A.A.; Murariu, D. Robotic versus Standard Harvest of Deep Inferior Epigastric Artery Perforator Flaps: Early Outcomes. *Plast. Reconstr. Surg. Glob. Open* **2022**, *10*, 64–65. [CrossRef]
34. Gkegkes, I.D.; Mamais, I.A.; Iavazzo, C. Robotics in general surgery: A systematic cost assessment. *J. Minim. Access. Surg.* **2017**, *13*, 243–255. [CrossRef] [PubMed]
35. Ahmed, K.; Ibrahim, A.; Wang, T.T.; Khan, N.; Challacombe, B.; Khan, M.S.; Dasgupta, P. Assessing the cost effectiveness of robotics in urological surgery—A systematic review. *BJU Int.* **2012**, *110*, 1544–1556. [CrossRef]
36. Iavazzo, C.; Gkegkes, I.D. Cost-benefit analysis of robotic surgery in gynaecological oncology. *Best. Pract. Res. Clin. Obstet. Gynaecol.* **2017**, *45*, 7–18. [CrossRef] [PubMed]
37. Donnely, E.; Griffin, M.F.; Butler, P.E. Robotic Surgery: A Novel Approach for Breast Surgery and Reconstruction. *Plast. Reconstr. Surg. Glob. Open* **2020**, *8*, e2578. [CrossRef]
38. Haddock, N.T.; Teotia, S.S. Efficient DIEP Flap: Bilateral Breast Reconstruction in Less Than Four Hours. *Plast. Reconstr. Surg. Glob. Open* **2021**, *9*, e3801. [CrossRef]

39. Jimenez, C.; Stanton, E.; Sung, C.; Wong, A.K. Does plastic surgery need a rewiring? A survey and systematic review on robotic-assisted surgery. *JPRAS Open* **2022**, *33*, 76–91. [CrossRef] [PubMed]
40. Barbon, C.; Grünherz, L.; Uyulmaz, S.; Giovanoli, P.; Lindenblatt, N. Exploring the learning curve of a new robotic microsurgical system for microsurgery. *JPRAS Open* **2022**, *34*, 126–133. [CrossRef]

Disclaimer/Publisher's Note: The statements, opinions and data contained in all publications are solely those of the individual author(s) and contributor(s) and not of MDPI and/or the editor(s). MDPI and/or the editor(s) disclaim responsibility for any injury to people or property resulting from any ideas, methods, instructions or products referred to in the content.

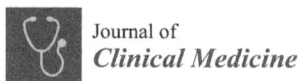

Article

The Controlling Nutritional Status (CONUT) Score for Prediction of Microvascular Flap Complications in Reconstructive Surgery

Rihards P. Rocans [1,2,*], Janis Zarins [3,4], Evita Bine [1], Renars Deksnis [5], Margarita Citovica [6], Simona Donina [7] and Biruta Mamaja [2]

1. Intensive Care Clinic, Riga East Clinical University Hospital, Hipokrata Street 2, LV-1079 Riga, Latvia; evitabine@gmail.com
2. Department of Anaesthesia and Intensive Care, Riga Stradins University, Dzirciema Street 16, LV-1007 Riga, Latvia; biruta.mamaja@aslimnica.lv
3. Department of Hand and Plastic Surgery, Microsurgery Centre of Latvia, Brivibas Street 410, LV-1024 Riga, Latvia; janis.zarins@mcl.lv
4. Baltic Biomaterials Centre of Excellence, Headquarters at Riga Technical University, Pulka Street 3, LV-1007 Riga, Latvia
5. Surgical Oncology Clinic, Riga East Clinical University Hospital, Hipokrata Street 4, LV-1079 Riga, Latvia; renars.deksnis@gmail.com
6. Laboratory Department, Riga East Clinical University Hospital, Hipokrata Street 2, LV-1079 Riga, Latvia; margarita.citovica@aslimnica.lv
7. Institute of Microbiology and Virology, Riga Stradins University, Ratsupites Street 5, LV-1067 Riga, Latvia; donsimon@inbox.lv
* Correspondence: rihards.rocans@gmail.com

Abstract: Microvascular flap surgery is a widely acknowledged procedure for significant defect reconstruction. Multiple flap complication risk factors have been identified, yet there are limited data on laboratory biomarkers for the prediction of flap loss. The controlling nutritional status (CONUT) score has demonstrated good postoperative outcome assessment ability in diverse surgical populations. We aim to assess the predictive value of the CONUT score for complications in microvascular flap surgery. This prospective cohort study includes 72 adult patients undergoing elective microvascular flap surgery. Preoperative blood draws for analysis of full blood count, total plasma cholesterol, and albumin concentrations were collected on the day of surgery before crystalloid infusion. Postoperative data on flap complications and duration of hospitalization were obtained. The overall complication rate was 15.2%. True flap loss with vascular compromise occurred in 5.6%. No differences in flap complications were found between different areas of reconstruction, anatomical flap types, or indications for surgery. Obesity was more common in patients with flap complications ($p = 0.01$). The CONUT score had an AUC of 0.813 (0.659–0.967, $p = 0.012$) for predicting complications other than true flap loss due to vascular compromise. A CONUT score > 2 was indicated as optimal during cut-off analysis ($p = 0.022$). Patients with flap complications had a longer duration of hospitalization (13.55, 10.99–16.11 vs. 25.38, 14.82–35.93; $p = 0.004$). Our findings indicate that the CONUT score has considerable predictive value in microvascular flap surgery.

Keywords: controlling nutritional status; microvascular flap complications; reconstructive surgery

Citation: Rocans, R.P.; Zarins, J.; Bine, E.; Deksnis, R.; Citovica, M.; Donina, S.; Mamaja, B. The Controlling Nutritional Status (CONUT) Score for Prediction of Microvascular Flap Complications in Reconstructive Surgery. *J. Clin. Med.* **2023**, *12*, 4794. https://doi.org/10.3390/jcm12144794

Academic Editor: Alexandre Bozec

Received: 6 June 2023
Revised: 14 July 2023
Accepted: 17 July 2023
Published: 20 July 2023

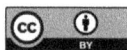

Copyright: © 2023 by the authors. Licensee MDPI, Basel, Switzerland. This article is an open access article distributed under the terms and conditions of the Creative Commons Attribution (CC BY) license (https://creativecommons.org/licenses/by/4.0/).

1. Introduction

Microvascular flap surgery has become a generally acknowledged procedure for significant defect reconstruction. Complex microvascular techniques and in-depth knowledge of blood rheology and microanastomosis function are required for this kind of surgery. Although substantial progress has been achieved in preventing complications, the rate of flap loss is still significant (1–7.1%) and can have significant adverse effects on the patient [1,2].

Flap thrombosis, flap hematoma, and flap loss are the most frequent and severe major surgical complications [3]. Mechanical problems comprise the most frequent causes of late flap failure (>48 h), and impaired arterial and venous blood supply is the most widespread cause of early flap failure (<48 h) [4]. Problematic and delayed healing, wound dehiscence, infection, fistula, and donor site problems are considered minor surgical complications. Even though microvascular flap transplantation relies on greatly specific surgical concepts, the issue of systemic reaction to surgical trauma and tissue healing is just as relevant here as in other types of surgery [5].

The most common indications for microvascular flap surgery are primary oncology or trauma, as well as defects related to previous surgery or infection [1]. Malnutrition may be common in patients requiring microvascular flap surgery [6], as many indications for microvascular flap surgery are also risk factors for poor nutritional status [7]. Previous studies show that the presence of malnutrition is a considerable risk factor for surgical complications in different patient populations [6–10]. Malnourished patients are at a higher risk of surgical complications such as wound dehiscence, infection, and fistula formation [9,11]. Most of these complications require reoperation, which can further increase patient morbidity and hospital costs [12]. Screening, assessing, and managing these patients is important because malnutrition is a modifiable pre-operative risk factor that, if addressed early, can reduce the risk of post-operative complications [13]. Given the complexity of microvascular flap transplantation and the availability of nutritional treatment strategies, a systematic approach to addressing nutrition risk significantly improves surgical outcomes in microvascular flap surgery [6,7].

The objective measurement of nutritional status can be performed with a wide range of tools, although there is no "gold standard" approach for measuring malnutrition [14]. The use of laboratory biomarkers for screening and assessing nutrition risk may be convenient, since laboratory evaluation is already routinely performed for preoperative assessment. Multiple studies have elucidated the link between laboratory biomarkers of poor nutritional status and surgical complications [6–8]. Studies have shown that lymphocyte count, albumin, prealbumin, and total plasma cholesterol are markers for poor nutritional status and can be quantified using nutritional assessment tools [15,16]. The controlling nutritional status (CONUT) score is an evolving tool that has demonstrated good postoperative outcome assessment ability in diverse surgical populations [9,17]. It is intended for inpatient assessment and is relatively simple to use, as it is calculated using only three values: serum albumin level, total cholesterol level, and total lymphocyte count [16]. A CONUT score of 0–1 is defined as no nutrition risk, and higher scores are defined as higher degrees of nutrition risk [16]. CONUT could be applied for assessment of nutrition risk in microvascular flap surgery due to its broad applicability and previous evidence for predicting complications in various surgical populations. The purpose of this study is to assess the predictive value of the CONUT score for predicting complications in elective microvascular flap surgery.

2. Materials and Methods

The study protocol and the informed consent form were approved by the Ethics Committee of Riga Stradins University (Approval Number 22-2/399/2021), and by the Science Department of Riga East University hospital (Approval Number Nr.AP/08-08/22/135).

2.1. Patient Selection

This prospective cohort study included 72 patients undergoing elective microvascular flap transplantation surgery at Riga East University Hospital from the 1 October 2021 to the 31 January 2023. Given the observational nature of our study, all surgical, anesthesia, and clinical management decisions were made by the attending physicians. The inclusion criterion was adult patients undergoing elective microvascular flap transplantation. The exclusion criteria were patients with sepsis or severe systemic bacterial infection; patients with autoimmune disorders; patients with blood-borne viral infections (Hepatitis B; Hepatitis C and HIV); pregnant patients and patients during lactation period; and patients with congenital hypercoagulability or any clotting disorder.

2.2. Anaesthesia and Surgical Protocol

All patients received general anesthesia (GA). Starting at the induction of anesthesia electrocardiography, pulse oximetry, noninvasive blood pressure, and end-tidal carbon dioxide concentration were monitored in all patients. Induction was performed using fentanyl (Fentanyl-Kalceks® 0.05 mg/mL, A/S Kalceks, Riga, Latvia) 1.5–2 µg/kg, and propofol (Propofol® 10 mg/mL, Fresenius Kabi AG, Bad Homburg, Germany) 1–2 mg/kg intravenously (iv). GA was maintained using sevoflurane (Sevorane®, AbbVie S.r.l., Campoverde, Italy) 0.8–1.2 MAC, and continuous analgesia was provided with fentanyl 1–1.5 µg/kg/h. Cisatracurium (Nimbex 2 mg/mL, Aspen Pharma Ltd., Dublin, Ireland) 0.15 mg/kg iv was used for tracheal intubation, followed by a continuous infusion of 1–2 µg/kg/min for muscle relaxation. Crystalloid infusion (RiLac, B. Braun Melsungen AG, Melsungen, Germany) was administered at a rate of 3.5 to 6.0 mL/kg iv per hour during surgery and the early postoperative period, with a target urine output of 1–2 mL/kg/h. Colloid fluid (Gelofusine, B. Braun Melsungen AG, Melsungen, Germany) was administered when an estimated blood loss of >500 mL occurred during surgery. Patients received both peripheral and central temperature monitoring during surgery to avoid hypothermia. Patients were administered vasopressors, such as ephedrine (Ephedrine Sintetica, Sintetica GmbH, Münster, Germany) or norepinephrine (Norepinephrine Sopharma, Sopharma AD, Sofia, Bulgaria), when their mean arterial blood pressure was below 65 mmHg for more than 5 min. Peripheral nerve blocks with ultrasound and neurostimulation guidance were performed when indicated. Patients received close postoperative monitoring of vital signs, fluid balance, and postoperative pain management in the post-anesthesia care unit. Postoperative thromboprophylaxis was provided with enoxaparin (Clexane®, Sanofi-Aventis S.A., Barcelona, Spain) 40 mg once daily from the first postoperative day for all patients. During and after surgery, patients with clinical symptoms of excessive blood loss or those with hemoglobin < 7 g/dL received blood product transfusions. All operations were performed by a team of highly experienced surgeons. The selection of flap type was based on the tissue type necessary for defect site reconstruction, the size of defect, the length of the pedicle, and the patient's positioning during surgery. The flaps used in the study were the anterolateral thigh flap, deep inferior epigastric artery perforator flap, fibular flap; radial free forearm flap, gracilis muscle flap, temporal artery flap, serratus anterior flap, latissimus dorsi flap, and medial condyle flap. The team of surgeons closely monitored the microvascular flap for the first five postoperative days. Flap patency was assessed using clinical assessment of flap color, temperature, tissue turgor, and capillary refill.

2.3. Data Collection

Blood draws were obtained on the day of surgery immediately upon the first arrival in the operating room before initiation of the first crystalloid infusion. Full blood count analysis was performed using the XN-1000 system (Sysmex Europe SE, Norderstedt, Germany). Concentrations of albumin were analyzed using the colorimetric method (Cobas C, Roche, Manheim, Germany). Concentrations of total plasma cholesterol were analyzed using the Enzymatic colorimetric method (Cobas C, Roche, Manheim, Germany). The serum albumin concentration, total peripheral lymphocyte count, and serum total cholesterol concentration were used to assign the CONUT score. As seen in Table 1, the CONUT score was determined by assigning laboratory values according to the tool first used by Ignacio de Ulíbarri and coauthors [16].

Table 1. The evaluation of the controlling nutritional status (CONUT) score; the controlling nutritional status (CONUT) score tool as first described by Ignacio de Ullibarri and coauthors [16].

Variable	Undernutrition Degree			
	Normal	Mild	Moderate	Severe
Serum albumin (g/dL)	≥3.50	3.00–3.49	2.50–2.99	<2.50
Score	0	2	4	6
Total lymphocyte count (/mm^3)	≥1600	1200–1599	800–1199	<800
Score	0	1	2	3
Total cholesterol (mg/dL)	≥180	140–179	100–139	<100
Score	0	1	2	3

Demographic data, comorbidities, data on perioperative course, anesthesia care, surgical outcome, length of stay in the intensive care unit (ICU), and total duration of hospitalization were obtained from written and electronic health records according to a previously defined protocol. Patients received postoperative daily follow up until discharge from the hospital.

2.4. Definitions

True flap loss was defined as flap blood supply deficiency due to arterial or venous anastomosis dysfunction or thrombosis that leads to complete loss of the transplanted flap. Other flap complications were defined as any of the following: hematoma (without interfering with flap blood supply), flap wound infection, secondary or incomplete flap wound healing, and partial flap loss. Partial flap loss was defined as the presence of distal marginal flap necrosis with no anastomosis dysfunction. Any flap complication was defined as the presence of either true flap loss or any other flap complication. ICU length of stay was the timing between admission to the ICU and discharge from the ICU to the ward. Hospital length of stay was the timing between admission to the hospital and discharge from the hospital.

2.5. Statistical Analysis

Statistical analysis was performed using SPSS Statistics for Windows, Version 26.0. (IBM Corp. Armonk, NY, USA). The Kolmogorov–Smirnov test was used to evaluate whether the datasets conformed to a normal distribution. Continuous variables conforming to normal distribution were presented as mean and CI95, while categorical variables were presented as median ± interquartile range (IQR). Differences in data distribution between the groups were evaluated using the Mann–Whitney U test for non-parametric datasets and the two-sample t-test or ANOVA for datasets conforming with normal distribution. A Chi-square test was applied for nominal variable sets. Binary logistic regression models were used to obtain odds ratios for specific variables. The receiver operator curve (ROC) and area under curve (AUC) were used for evaluating the diagnostic ability of a binary classifier system. Youden's Index (YI) and the Concordance Probability Method (CZ) was used for defining optimal cut-off values [18]. Statistical significance was assumed if two-tailed $p < 0.05$.

3. Results

In total, 72 patients—40 (55.6%) men and 32 (44.4%) women—were included. The mean age was 55.3 years (95% CI95 51.5–59.1). The overall complication rate was 15.2% ($n = 11$). True flap loss with vascular compromise occurred in 5.6% ($n = 4$), with two of these cases being late flap loss (>72 h). Both cases of early true flap loss underwent urgent anastomosis revision. Both cases of late flap loss underwent repeated elective microvascular flap transplantation. Other flap complications occurred in seven cases, with difficult flap healing or partial flap loss occurring in 5.6% ($n = 4$), flap infection occurring in one, and hematoma occurring in two cases. The median number of revisions in patients with true flap loss was 1.5 (IQR 1). The median number of revisions in patients with other flap complications was 1 (IQR 0.75, p = 0.223).

As seen in Table 2, there were no significant differences in age or gender distribution in patients with any flap complications or flap loss, and in patients without complications. No significant differences in true flap failure or other flap complications were found between different areas of reconstruction and different anatomical flap types. No significant differences in true flap failure or other flap complications were found between different indications for reconstruction. Of the included comorbidities, obesity was found to be more common in patients with any flap complications (p = 0.01). Only two patients had a BMI < 20 kg/m^2, and there was no statistically significant link between decreased BMI and any flap complications. No statistically significant link was found between BMI and CONUT score. No significant differences in the rates of true flap failure or other flap complications were found in patients with other comorbidities.

Table 2. Demographic characteristics, surgical considerations, and comorbidities; data are presented as mean (CI95) or count (percentage). Abbreviations—BMI (body mass index); ENT (ear, nose, and throat surgery); DIEP (deep inferior epigastric artery perforator flap); ALT (anterolateral thigh flap).

Patient Group	Overall n = 72	No Complications n = 61	True Flap Loss n = 4	Any Flap Complications n = 11	p-Value
Demographical data					
Mean age, years	55.3 (51.5–59.1)	56.9 (61.0–65.4)	65.0 (63.5–66.5)	49.6 (37.7–56.1)	0.057
Sex (female), n (%)	32 (44.4%)	25 (40.1%)	2 (50.0%)	5 (45.5%)	0.418
Area of reconstruction					
Extremity, n (%)	15 (20.8%)	12 (19.6%)	-	3 (27.3%)	0.289
ENT, n (%)	26 (36.1%)	22 (36.1%)	2 (50.0%)	4 (36.4%)	0.496
Head and neck, n (%)	16 (22.2%)	14 (30.0%)	1 (25.0%)	2 (18.2%)	0.322
Breast, n (%)	15 (20.8%)	13 (21.3%)	1 (25.0%)	2 (18.2%)	0.457
Microvascular flap type					
ALT, (%)	32 (44.4%)	27 (44.3%)	2 (50.0%)	5 (45.5%)	0.828
Fibular flap, (%)	9 (12.5%)	8 (13.1%)	1 (25.0%)	1 (9.1%)	0.478
DIEP, n (%)	9 (12.5%)	7 (11.5%)	-	2 (18.2%)	0.528
Radial artery flap, n (%)	6 (8.3%)	6 (9.8%)	-	-	-
Other, n (%)	16 (22.2%)	13 (21.3%)	1 (25.0%)	3 (27.3%)	0.413
Indication for surgery					
Trauma, n (%)	8 (11.1%)	6 (10.1%)	-	1 (9.1%)	0.918
Oncology, n (%)	40 (55.6%)	32 (58.2%)	3 (75.0%)	6 (54.5%)	0.469
Defect, n (%)	19 (26.4%)	11 (20.0%)	1 (25.0%)	4 (36.4%)	0.511
Infection, n (%)	5 (6.9%)	5 (8.2%)	-	-	-
Comorbidities					
Coronary artery disease, n (%)	4 (5.6%)	3 (4.9%)	1 (25.0%)	1 (9.1%)	0.059
Diabetes mellitus, n (%)	5 (6.9%)	4 (6.6%)	-	1 (9.1%)	0.691
Hypertension, n (%)	28 (38.8%)	19 (31.1%)	3 (75.0%)	6 (54.5%)	0.133
Dyslipidemia, n (%)	16 (22.2%)	13 (21.3%)	1 (25.0%)	3 (27.3%)	0.624
Smoking history, n (%)	13 (18.1%)	11 (18.0%)	1 (25.0%)	2 (18.2%)	0.249
Obesity (BMI > 30 kg/m^2), n (%)	12 (16.6%)	8 (13.1%)	2 (50.0%)	5 (45.5%)	0.010 **
Cerebrovascular accident, n (%)	4 (5.6%)	4 (6.6%)	-	-	0.620

The ** symbol is used to indicate statistical significance when comparing the group without complications to both the true flap loss group and the any flap complications group.

As seen in Table 3, no significant links were found between the duration of surgery and anesthesia factors and any flap complications. A higher intraoperative hematocrit was associated with flap complications, with the highest intraoperative hematocrit found in cases with subsequent true flap loss (p = 0.009). Only one patient received intraoperative hemotransfusion, and five patients received hemotransfusion in the early postoperative period. There was no significant link between the presence of hemotransfusion and any flap complications.

Table 3. Intraoperative and anesthesia considerations; data are presented as mean (CI95) or count (percentage).

Patient Group	Overall $n = 72$	No Complications $n = 61$	True Flap Loss $n = 4$	Any Flap Complications $n = 11$	p-Value
Duration of surgery, hours	6.39 (5.75–7.02)	6.33 (5.59–7.07)	7.63 (5.86–9.39)	6.66 (5.29–8.04)	0.235
Volume of intraoperative crystalloid, mL	2345.83 (2141.39–2550.28)	2352.50 (2133.31–2571.69)	2875.00 (1681.58–4068.42)	2312.50 (1608.14–3016.86)	0.145
Volume of intraoperative colloid, mL	506.25 (401.74–610.76)	482.50 (367.10–597.90)	500.00 (-)	625.00 (329.42–920.58)	0.471
Intraoperative colloid to crystalloid ratio	0.22 (0.17–0.27)	0.20 (0.15–0.25)	0.18 (0.10–0.27)	0.33 (0.09–0.56)	0.306
Intraoperative hematocrit, %	30.60 (29.20–32.00)	29.58 (27.70–31.45)	31.50 (25.15–37.85)	34.40 (30.32–38.48)	0.009 *
Use of vasopressors/sympathomimetics, n (%)	41 (56.90%)	36 (59.00%)	2 (50.00%)	6 (54.50%)	0.549

The * symbol is used to indicate statistical significance when comparing the group without complications to the any flap complications group.

As seen in Table 4, patients with any flap complications had a significantly lower plasma lymphocyte count ($p = 0.001$). Multivariate regression analysis revealed that an increase in lymphocyte count decreases the incidence of all complications (OR 0.998 CI95 0.996–0.999). Patients with any flap complications had a significantly lower plasma monocyte count ($p = 0.021$). No differences in plasma lymphocyte/monocyte ratio, plasma albumin, and total plasma cholesterol were found in patients with any flap complications.

Table 4. Biomarkers and nutritional systems for predicting any flap complications; data are presented as mean (CI95), median (IQR), or count (percentage).

Patient Group	Overall $n = 72$	No Complications $n = 61$	Any Flap Complications $n = 11$	p-Value
Biomarkers				
Lymphocyte count 10^9/L	1.59 (1.39–1.79)	1.71 (1.49–1.92)	0.97 (0.67–1.26)	0.001 *
Monocyte count 10^9/L	0.55 (0.48–0.62)	0.58 (0.51–0.66)	0.37 (0.22–0.51)	0.021 *
Lymphocyte/monocyte ratio	3.46 (2.91–4.02)	3.55 (2.90–4.20)	2.97 (2.28–3.65)	0.830
Mean plasma albumin, g/dL	3.94 (3.81–4.06)	3.96 (3.84–4.09)	3.79 (3.28–4.30)	0.631
Mean total plasma cholesterol, mg/dL	196.58 (185.21–207.95)	198.44 (186.43–210.45)	186.73 (147.93–225.53)	0.310
Nutritional assessment systems				
CONUT score	2(2)	2 (3)	3 (6)	0.013 *
CONUT ≤ 2	50 (69.4%)	46 (75.4%)	4 (36.4%)	0.009 *

The * symbol is used to indicate statistical significance when comparing the group without complications to the any flap complications group.

As seen in Figure 1, analysis on the predictive accuracy of CONUT score of other surgical complications found that CONUT score had an AUC of 0.813 (0.659–0.967, $p = 0.012$). A CONUT score of >2 was found to be optimal during cut-off analysis (Sensitivity 21.1%, Specificity 95.6%, PPV 66.7%, NPV 74.1%, $p = 0.022$). CONUT score of >2 increases the odds of other flap complications (OR 5.4, CI95 1.38–20.90, $p = 0.015$). Univariate regression revealed that any increase in CONUT score increased the odds of other flap complications (OR 1.43 1.09–1.85). Patients with any flap complications had a longer duration of hospitalization (13.55, 10.99–16.11 vs. 25.38, 14.82–35.93; $p = 0.004$). There was no difference in duration of ICU stay between patients with flap complications and patients with no flap complications (1.13, 0.03–2.26 vs. 1.50 1.00–2.00, $p = 0.471$).

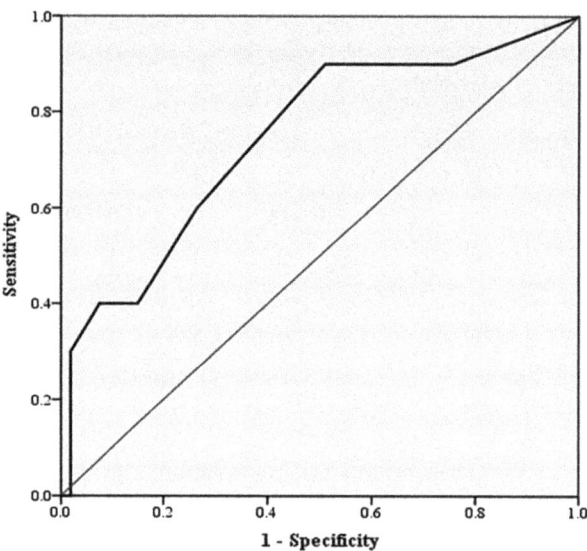

Figure 1. ROC curve characteristics of CONUT score for predicting complications in microvascular flap surgery; receiver operator curve characteristics and area under curve of CONUT score for predicting the presence of flap complications other than true flap loss. CONUT scores had an AUC of 0.813 (CI95 0.659–0.967, $p = 0.012$).

4. Discussion

The main findings of the present study were that an increase in the preoperative CONUT index is a reliable predictor for flap complications, with a CONUT score of >2 being the optimal cut-off for predicting complication risk. Flap complications were found to be linked to lymphocytopenia, monocytopenia, hematocrit, and obesity. The incidence of true flap loss was 6.2%, and the incidence of other less severe complications was 9.2%. The duration of hospitalization was significantly longer in patients who had flap complications.

Microvascular flap transplantation requires complex microvascular techniques, and flap success relies on the function of microanastomosis and adequate flap perfusion [4]. While these are greatly specific concepts, the issue of systemic reaction to surgical trauma and tissue healing and nutrition is just as relevant here as in other types of surgery [5]. Malnourished patients are more likely to experience complications during and after surgery, longer hospital stays, and a slower recovery time both in the general surgical population [8–10] and in microvascular flap surgery [6,7]. Given the complexity of the procedure and severity of the complications, clinical prediction tools regarding nutrition risk may be used during preoperative assessments to identify patients who may require more extensive evaluation or preparation before surgery [6,7]. A study by Yu and co-authors suggests that the prognostic nutritional index (PNI), a score including some of the same parameters as CONUT, can be simply and effectively used to predict free flap failure in extremity reconstruction [6]. Our results indicate that an increased CONUT score significantly increases the odds of postoperative complications. To the best of our knowledge, no previous studies have elucidated the predictive value of CONUT in microvascular flap surgery. However, our findings coincide with data from different surgical populations wherein CONUT has been shown to reliably predict complications and mortality [8,19]. Additionally, our results suggest that patients with flap complications had longer hospital stays. This coincides with previous studies that report longer hospital stays and increased hospital costs in patients who experience free flap failure in breast and head and neck reconstruction [20,21]. Considering that any increase in the CONUT score increases the risk of flap complications it can also consequently lead to longer hospital stays and increased costs.

In our study, we found CONUT > 2 to be the most optimal cut-off value, which also coincides with some data from previous studies in other surgical populations [9,17,22]. It must be noted that we found a CONUT > 2 cut-off value to have a relatively low sensitivity (21.1%) and a high specificity (95.6%). These results imply that a cut-off value of CONUT > 2 is best utilized for excluding patients who are at a low nutrition risk and low risk of subsequent flap complications.

Interestingly, while our data showed CONUT to be a reliable predictor for flap complications, it was not a reliable predictor specifically for true flap loss. This indicates that the pathophysiology of true flap loss due to anastomosis compromise [23] may be separate from the pathophysiology of other surgical complications in microvascular flap surgery. Most minor complications in microvascular flap surgery, such as wound dehiscence, infection, and fistula formation, occur due to inadequate tissue healing and regeneration [24]. These complications may be linked to undernutrition [7] instead of being a direct result of early anastomosis compromise. Notably, even minor complications place the patient at an increased risk of re-exploration or repeated microvascular flap transplantation [25]. Furthermore, patients receiving microvascular flap transplantation are predisposed to difficult wound healing, both at the site of reconstruction and at the donor site [25].

Plasma lymphocyte count is a component of CONUT that may have a substantial role in the pathophysiology of microvascular flap complications. Studies in various surgical populations show that patients with preoperative lymphocytopenia had a significantly higher incidence of complications compared to those with a normal lymphocyte level at admission [5,26,27]. Lymphocyte recovery in the first postoperative days could play an important role in the mechanisms of tissue repair, and a primary role in wound healing [28]. Monocytes are the most responsive leukocytes in response to trauma [29] and multiple monocyte immunophenotypic alterations are observed upon surgery [30,31]. In contrast to our findings, Kosec and co-authors did not find a link between preoperative monocyte count and postoperative complications in microvascular flap surgery [5].

Multiple patient-related risk factors, including coronary artery disease, diabetes, smoking, peripheral arterial vascular disease, arterial hypertension, and higher ASA score, are related to flap failure [1]. Obesity has been deemed to be a risk factor for poor surgical outcomes in medical care, but the majority of published studies in various surgical populations have been uncertain [32–34]. Some previous studies found obesity to be associated with increased perioperative risk in free abdominally based autologous breast reconstruction, which coincides with our findings [35,36]. Conversely, multiple studies have also evidenced that obesity does not increase the risk of postoperative complications in microvascular flap surgery [37–39]. However, it must be noted that the presence of obesity does not exclude the presence of double-burden malnutrition, which can also have detrimental effects on overall health [40,41]. Furthermore, the study by Ignacio de Ulíbarri and coauthors found no relationship between BMI and undernutrition in their study population, as BMI is not a reliable indicator for acute malnutrition [16]. Our data indicate that both obesity and nutrition risk increase the rate of flap complications, which indicates that both conditions should be assessed and treated to improve outcomes in microvascular flap surgery.

This study had several limitations. Firstly, given the observational nature of our study, individual surgical, anesthesia, and nutritional management decision-making was performed by the clinicians, and may have varied between cases. Secondly, ours was a single-center study, which affects the possible generalizability of the findings. Notably, a considerable part of our study population has oncology as a primary diagnosis, which likely introduces additional confounding risk factors for surgical complications. Conversely, it must be noted that patients with oncology as a primary diagnosis are very likely to benefit from an assessment of nutrition risk [8,9,15,17]. It should be noted that the presence of radiotherapy, which can present confounding factors, was not considered in this study. Finally, it is important to note that serum albumin, which is an important item in both the CONUT and PNI scores, is not a part of current definitions of malnutrition [42]. Therefore, CONUT score results are considered to be indicators of nutrition risk rather than an assessment of nutritional status. Further studies are needed to clarify the use of nutrition risk assessment tools to predict complications in different patient populations, and to specify the use of specific nutritional interventions to improve outcomes in microvascular flap surgery.

5. Conclusions

Assessment of nutritional risk to estimate the risk of microvascular flap complications using the CONUT score has considerable predictive value. Patients undergoing this type of surgery can be evaluated in terms of predicting nutritional risk to optimize decision-making in perioperative care.

Author Contributions: R.P.R., B.M., S.D. and M.C. conceived and planned the study. J.Z., R.P.R., R.D. and M.C. participated in data collection. R.P.R. and E.B. performed data curation and statistical analysis. R.P.R., J.Z., B.M., S.D. and E.B. interpreted the results and prepared the draft. All authors have read and agreed to the published version of the manuscript.

Funding: The authors declare that Riga Stradiņš University kindly covered the publication fee for this article (Grant Reference Number 6-DN-20/2/2023). The funder was not involved in the study design, collection, analysis, interpretation of data or writing of this article.

Institutional Review Board Statement: The study protocol and the informed consent form were approved by the Ethics Committee of Riga Stradins University (Approval Number 22-2/399/2021; Approval date 8 July 2021), and by the Science Department of Riga East University Hospital (Approval Number AP/08-08/22/135; Approval date 8 November 2022).

Informed Consent Statement: Informed consent was obtained from all subjects involved in the study.

Data Availability Statement: The datasets used and analyzed during the current study are available from the corresponding author upon reasonable request. The corresponding author will ensure individual privacy is not compromised during the transfer of datasets.

Acknowledgments: We would like to acknowledge the help of Vita Kalnberzina, Department of English studies, University of Latvia, for reviewing and revising this manuscript's English grammar and syntax.

Conflicts of Interest: The authors declare no conflict of interest.

References

1. Lese, I.; Biedermann, R.; Constantinescu, M.; Grobbelaar, A.O.; Olariu, R. Predicting risk factors that lead to free flap failure and vascular compromise: A single unit experience with 565 free tissue transfers. *J. Plast. Reconstr. Aesthet. Surg.* **2021**, *74*, 512–522. [CrossRef] [PubMed]
2. Hanasono, M.M.; Butler, C.E. Prevention and treatment of thrombosis in microvascular surgery. *J. Reconstr. Microsurg.* **2008**, *24*, 305–314. [CrossRef] [PubMed]
3. Lo, S.L.; Yen, Y.H.; Lee, P.J.; Liu, C.C.; Pu, C.M. Factors Influencing Postoperative Complications in Reconstructive Microsurgery for Head and Neck Cancer. *J. Oral Maxillofac. Surg.* **2017**, *75*, 867–873. [CrossRef]
4. Novakovic, D.; Patel, R.S.; Goldstein, D.P.; Gullane, P.J. Salvage of failed free flaps used in head and neck reconstruction. *Head Neck Oncol.* **2009**, *1*, 33. [CrossRef] [PubMed]
5. Košec, A.; Solter, D.; Ribić, A.; Knežević, M.; Vagić, D.; Pegan, A. Systemic Inflammatory Markers as Predictors of Postoperative Complications and Survival in Patients with Advanced Head and Neck Squamous Cell Carcinoma Undergoing Free-Flap Reconstruction. *J. Oral Maxillofac. Surg.* **2022**, *80*, 744–755. [CrossRef] [PubMed]
6. Yu, J.; Hong, J.P.; Suh, H.P.; Park, J.Y.; Kim, D.H.; Ha, S.; Lee, J.; Hwang, J.H.; Kim, Y.K. Prognostic Nutritional Index is a Predictor of Free Flap Failure in Extremity Reconstruction. *Nutrients* **2020**, *12*, 562. [CrossRef]
7. Shum, J.; Markiewicz, M.R.; Park, E.; Bui, T.; Lubek, J.; Bell, R.B.; Dierks, E.J. Low prealbumin level is a risk factor for microvascular free flap failure. *J. Oral Maxillofac. Surg.* **2014**, *72*, 169–177. [CrossRef]
8. Takagi, K.; Domagala, P.; Polak, W.G.; Buettner, S.; Wijnhoven, B.P.L.; Ijzermans, J.N.M. Prognostic significance of the controlling nutritional status (CONUT) score in patients undergoing gastrectomy for gastric cancer: A systematic review and meta-analysis. *BMC Surg.* **2019**, *19*, 129. [CrossRef]
9. Qian, Y.; Liu, H.; Pan, J.; Yu, W.; Lv, J.; Yan, J.; Gao, J.; Wang, X.; Ge, X.; Zhou, W. Preoperative Controlling Nutritional Status (CONUT) score predicts short-term outcomes of patients with gastric cancer after laparoscopy-assisted radical gastrectomy. *World J. Surg. Oncol.* **2021**, *19*, 25. [CrossRef]

10. Venianaki, M.; Andreou, A.; Nikolouzakis, T.K.; Chrysos, E.; Chalkiadakis, G.; Lasithiotakis, K. Factors Associated with Malnutrition and Its Impact on Postoperative Outcomes in Older Patients. *J. Clin. Med.* **2021**, *10*, 2550. [CrossRef]
11. Abela, G. The potential benefits and harms of early feeding post-surgery: A literature review. *Int. Wound J.* **2017**, *14*, 870–873. [CrossRef]
12. Jones, N.F.; Jarrahy, R.; Song, J.I.; Kaufman, M.R.; Markowitz, B. Postoperative medical complications—Not microsurgical complications—Negatively influence the morbidity, mortality, and true costs after microsurgical reconstruction for head and neck cancer. *Plast. Reconstr. Surg.* **2007**, *119*, 2053–2060. [CrossRef]
13. Jie, B.; Jiang, Z.M.; Nolan, M.T.; Zhu, S.N.; Yu, K.; Kondrup, J. Impact of preoperative nutritional support on clinical outcome in abdominal surgical patients at nutritional risk. *Nutrition* **2012**, *28*, 1022–1027. [CrossRef]
14. Skipper, A.; Coltman, A.; Tomesko, J.; Charney, P.; Porcari, J.; Piemonte, T.A.; Cheng, F.W. Adult Malnutrition (Undernutrition) Screening: An Evidence Analysis Center Systematic Review. *J. Acad. Nutr. Diet.* **2020**, *120*, 669–708. [CrossRef]
15. Smale, B.F.; Mullen, J.L.; Buzby, G.P.; Rosato, E.F. The efficacy of nutritional assessment and support in cancer surgery. *Cancer* **1981**, *47*, 2375–2381. [CrossRef]
16. de Ulíbarri, J.I.; González-Madroño, A.; de Villar, N.G.; González, P.; González, B.; Mancha, A.; Rodríguez, F.; Fernández, G. CONUT: A tool for controlling nutritional status. First validation in a hospital population. *Nutr. Hosp.* **2005**, *20*, 38–45.
17. Toyokawa, T.; Kubo, N.; Tamura, T.; Sakurai, K.; Amano, R.; Tanaka, H.; Muguruma, K.; Yashiro, M.; Hirakawa, K.; Ohira, M. The pretreatment Controlling Nutritional Status (CONUT) score is an independent prognostic factor in patients with resectable thoracic esophageal squamous cell carcinoma: Results from a retrospective study. *BMC Cancer* **2016**, *16*, 722. [CrossRef]
18. Unal, I. Defining an Optimal Cut-Point Value in ROC Analysis: An Alternative Approach. *Comput. Math. Methods Med.* **2017**, *2017*, 3762651. [CrossRef]
19. Lee, S.C.; Lee, J.G.; Lee, S.H.; Kim, E.Y.; Chang, J.; Kim, D.J.; Paik, H.C.; Chung, K.Y.; Jung, J.Y. Prediction of postoperative pulmonary complications using preoperative controlling nutritional status (CONUT) score in patients with resectable non-small cell lung cancer. *Sci. Rep.* **2020**, *10*, 12385. [CrossRef]
20. Lindeborg, M.M.; Sethi, R.K.V.; Puram, S.V.; Parikh, A.; Yarlagadda, B.; Varvares, M.; Emerick, K.; Lin, D.; Durand, M.L.; Deschler, D.G. Predicting length of stay in head and neck patients who undergo free flap reconstruction. *Laryngoscope Investig. Otolaryngol.* **2020**, *5*, 461–467. [CrossRef]
21. O'Neill, A.C.; Mughal, M.; Saggaf, M.M.; Wisniewski, A.; Zhong, T.; Hofer, S.O.P. A structured pathway for accelerated postoperative recovery reduces hospital stay and cost of care following microvascular breast reconstruction without increased complications. *J. Plast. Reconstr. Aesthet. Surg.* **2020**, *73*, 19–26. [CrossRef] [PubMed]
22. Iseki, Y.; Shibutani, M.; Maeda, K.; Nagahara, H.; Ohtani, H.; Sugano, K.; Ikeya, T.; Muguruma, K.; Tanaka, H.; Toyokawa, T.; et al. Impact of the Preoperative Controlling Nutritional Status (CONUT) Score on the Survival after Curative Surgery for Colorectal Cancer. *PLoS ONE* **2015**, *10*, e0132488. [CrossRef] [PubMed]
23. Adams, J.; Charlton, P. Anaesthesia for microvascular free tissue transfer. *BJA CEPD Rev.* **2003**, *3*, 33–37. [CrossRef]
24. Felekis, D.; Eleftheriadou, A.; Papadakos, G.; Bosinakou, I.; Ferekidou, E.; Kandiloros, D.; Katsaragakis, S.; Charalabopoulos, K.; Manolopoulos, L. Effect of perioperative immuno-enhanced enteral nutrition on inflammatory response, nutritional status, and outcomes in head and neck cancer patients undergoing major surgery. *Nutr. Cancer* **2010**, *62*, 1105–1112. [CrossRef] [PubMed]
25. Pohlenz, P.; Klatt, J.; Schön, G.; Blessmann, M.; Li, L.; Schmelzle, R. Microvascular free flaps in head and neck surgery: Complications and outcome of 1000 flaps. *Int. J. Oral Maxillofac. Surg.* **2012**, *41*, 739–743. [CrossRef]
26. Chiarelli, M.; Achilli, P.; Tagliabue, F.; Brivio, A.; Airoldi, A.; Guttadauro, A.; Porro, F.; Fumagalli, L. Perioperative lymphocytopenia predicts mortality and severe complications after intestinal surgery. *Ann. Transl. Med.* **2019**, *7*, 311. [CrossRef]
27. Lee, Y.Y.; Choi, C.H.; Sung, C.O.; Do, I.G.; Hub, S.J.; Kim, H.J.; Kim, T.J.; Lee, J.W.; Bae, D.S.; Kim, B.G. Clinical significance of changes in peripheral lymphocyte count after surgery in early cervical cancer. *Gynecol. Oncol.* **2012**, *127*, 107–113. [CrossRef]
28. Vulliamy, P.E.; Perkins, Z.B.; Brohi, K.; Manson, J. Persistent lymphopenia is an independent predictor of mortality in critically ill emergency general surgical patients. *Eur. J. Trauma Emerg. Surg.* **2016**, *42*, 755–760. [CrossRef]
29. Chen, T.; Delano, M.J.; Chen, K.; Sperry, J.L.; Namas, R.A.; Lamparello, A.J.; Deng, M.; Conroy, J.; Moldawer, L.L.; Efron, P.A.; et al. A road map from single-cell transcriptome to patient classification for the immune response to trauma. *JCI Insight* **2021**, *6*, e145108. [CrossRef]
30. Edomskis, P.P.; Dik, W.A.; Sparreboom, C.L.; Nagtzaam, N.M.A.; van Oudenaren, A.; Lambrichts, D.P.V.; Bayon, Y.; van Dongen, N.N.N.; Menon, A.G.; de Graaf, E.J.R.; et al. Monocyte response after colorectal surgery: A prospective cohort study. *Front. Immunol.* **2022**, *13*, 1031216. [CrossRef]
31. Klava, A.; Windsor, A.; Boylston, A.W.; Reynolds, J.V.; Ramsden, C.W.; Guillou, P.J. Monocyte activation after open and laparoscopic surgery. *Br. J. Surg.* **1997**, *84*, 1152–1156.
32. Malietzis, G.; Johns, N.; Al-Hassi, H.O.; Knight, S.C.; Kennedy, R.H.; Fearon, K.C.; Aziz, O.; Jenkins, J.T. Low Muscularity and Myosteatosis Is Related to the Host Systemic Inflammatory Response in Patients Undergoing Surgery for Colorectal Cancer. *Ann. Surg.* **2016**, *263*, 320–325. [CrossRef]
33. Pedrazzani, C.; Conti, C.; Zamboni, G.A.; Chincarini, M.; Turri, G.; Valdegamberi, A.; Guglielmi, A. Impact of visceral obesity and sarcobesity on surgical outcomes and recovery after laparoscopic resection for colorectal cancer. *Clin. Nutr.* **2020**, *39*, 3763–3770. [CrossRef]
34. Ri, M.; Aikou, S.; Seto, Y. Obesity as a surgical risk factor. *Ann. Gastroenterol. Surg.* **2017**, *2*, 13–21. [CrossRef]

35. Fischer, J.P.; Nelson, J.A.; Sieber, B.; Cleveland, E.; Kovach, S.J.; Wu, L.C.; Serletti, J.M.; Kanchwala, S. Free tissue transfer in the obese patient: An outcome and cost analysis in 1258 consecutive abdominally based reconstructions. *Plast. Reconstr. Surg.* **2013**, *131*, 681e–692e. [CrossRef]
36. Sinha, S.; Ruskin, O.; D'Angelo, A.; McCombe, D.; Morrison, W.A.; Webb, A. Are overweight and obese patients who receive autologous free-flap breast reconstruction satisfied with their postoperative outcome? A single-centre study. *J. Plast. Reconstr. Aesthet. Surg.* **2016**, *69*, 30–36. [CrossRef]
37. Chang, E.I.; Liu, J. Prospective Evaluation of Obese Patients Undergoing Autologous Abdominal Free Flap Breast Reconstruction. *Plast. Reconstr. Surg.* **2018**, *142*, 120e–125e. [CrossRef]
38. de la Garza, G.; Militsakh, O.; Panwar, A.; Galloway, T.L.; Jorgensen, J.B.; Ledgerwood, L.G.; Kaiser, K.; Kitzerow, C.; Shnayder, Y.; Neumann, C.A.; et al. Obesity and perioperative complications in head and neck free tissue reconstruction. *Head Neck* **2016**, *38* (Suppl. S1), E1188–E1191. [CrossRef]
39. Crippen, M.M.; Brady, J.S.; Mozeika, A.M.; Eloy, J.A.; Baredes, S.; Park, R.C.W. Impact of Body Mass Index on Operative Outcomes in Head and Neck Free Flap Surgery. *Otolaryngol. Head Neck Surg.* **2018**, *159*, 817–823. [CrossRef]
40. Popkin, B.M.; Corvalan, C.; Grummer-Strawn, L.M. Dynamics of the double burden of malnutrition and the changing nutrition reality. *Lancet* **2020**, *395*, 65–74. [CrossRef]
41. Wells, J.C.; Sawaya, A.L.; Wibaek, R.; Mwangome, M.; Poullas, M.S.; Yajnik, C.S.; Demaio, A. The double burden of malnutrition: Aetiological pathways and consequences for health. *Lancet* **2020**, *395*, 75–88. [CrossRef] [PubMed]
42. Evans, D.C.; Corkins, M.R.; Malone, A.; Miller, S.; Mogensen, K.M.; Guenter, P. The Use of Visceral Proteins as Nutrition Markers: An ASPEN Position Paper. *Nutr. Clin. Pract.* **2021**, *36*, 22–28. [CrossRef] [PubMed]

Disclaimer/Publisher's Note: The statements, opinions and data contained in all publications are solely those of the individual author(s) and contributor(s) and not of MDPI and/or the editor(s). MDPI and/or the editor(s) disclaim responsibility for any injury to people or property resulting from any ideas, methods, instructions or products referred to in the content.

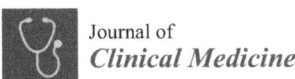

Article

What Is the Minimum Number of Sutures for Microvascular Anastomosis during Replantation?

Hyung-suk Yi [†], Byeong-seok Kim [†], Yoon-soo Kim, Jin-hyung Park and Hong-il Kim *

Department of Plastic and Reconstructive Surgery, Kosin University Gospel Hospital,
Kosin University College of Medicine, Busan 49267, Republic of Korea
* Correspondence: immtkg4u@daum.net; Tel.: +82-51-990-6131
† These authors contributed equally to this work.

Abstract: As vessel diameter decreases, reperfusion after anastomosis becomes more difficult. When a blood vessel is sutured, its inner diameter becomes narrower owing to the thickness of the suture material and the number of sutures. To minimize this, we attempted replantation using a 2-point suture technique. We reviewed cases of arterial anastomosis in vessels with a diameter of less than 0.3 mm during replantation performed over a four-year period. In all cases, close observation was followed by absolute bed rest. If reperfusion was not achieved, a tie-over dressing was applied, and hyperbaric oxygen therapy was administered in the form of a composite graft. Of the 21 replantation cases, 19 were considered successful. Furthermore, the 2-point suture technique was performed in 12 cases, of which 11 survived. When three or four sutures were performed in nine patients, eight of these cases survived. Composite graft conversion was found in three cases in which the 2-point suture technique was used, and two of these cases survived. The survival rate was high in cases where 2-point sutures were used, and there were few cases of conversion to a composite graft. Reducing the number of sutures aids in optimizing reperfusion.

Keywords: reconstructive surgical procedures; microsurgery; suture technique; skin grafting

1. Introduction

Accurate and successful microvascular anastomosis is essential for free tissue transfer and limb replantation [1]. Despite advancements in microsurgical instruments and techniques, microvascular anastomosis is challenging and requires advanced microsurgical techniques [2,3]. Achieving accurate approximation of anastomosed vessels, eversion of the vessel ends, and proper contact of the intimal layers with no uneven leading points for thrombosis are essential for a successful anastomosis. The conventional technique of microvascular anastomosis with several interrupted sutures is a well-proven method; however, it is still imperfect. Due to the high number of stitches, the technique is time-consuming and increases the ischemia time [4]. Moreover, small blood vessels of 0.3 mm or less at the level of supermicrosurgery do not have a constant location, so it takes a lot of time to find suitable blood vessels in trauma situations [4]. Additionally, a forceps and thin thread suitable for supermicrosugery are required, but if there is no such tool and there is little clinical experience, it takes a lot of time. Also, the stitching procedure causes surgical trauma, and the suture material acts as a foreign body in the lumen, which could lead to thrombosis [5,6]. Therefore, to reduce the surgical time and exposure to suture materials, research on reducing the number of sutures and novel suturing techniques is ongoing [7–11]. Recently, a study showed that anastomosis is possible with three stitches at an angle of 120° [12,13]. In this study, the authors introduced a 2-point suture technique with an angle of 180° to reduce vascular occlusive complications caused by stitches while ensuring lumen eversion. This technique can be used in cases where there is little supermicrosurgery experience or the instrument required for supermicrosurgery is insufficient (e.g., superfine

Citation: Yi, H.-s.; Kim, B.-s.; Kim, Y.-s.; Park, J.-h.; Kim, H.-i. What Is the Minimum Number of Sutures for Microvascular Anastomosis during Replantation? *J. Clin. Med.* **2023**, *12*, 2891. https://doi.org/10.3390/jcm12082891

Academic Editor: Albert H. Chao

Received: 24 February 2023
Revised: 9 April 2023
Accepted: 14 April 2023
Published: 15 April 2023

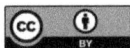

Copyright: © 2023 by the authors. Licensee MDPI, Basel, Switzerland. This article is an open access article distributed under the terms and conditions of the Creative Commons Attribution (CC BY) license (https://creativecommons.org/licenses/by/4.0/).

tip forceps or 11-0 or 12-0 sutures). The objective of this study was to evaluate the feasibility, speed, and reliability of this new technique and contribute to ongoing efforts to improve microvascular anastomosis.

2. Materials and Methods

2.1. Patients Selection and Study Design

From January 2017 to December 2021, the medical records of patients who underwent arterial anastomosis of vessels that were less than 0.3 mm in diameter during replantation at our institution were retrospectively reviewed. Electronic medical records, X-ray films, clinical photographs of the wounds, and demographic information were reviewed. Patient characteristics, preoperative assessments, and operative data (e.g., number of stitches and anastomosis) were recorded. The recorded patient data included age, sex, body mass index, level of the injury, the mechanism of the injury, comorbid medical conditions, anticoagulant use, and tobacco use. We categorized the mechanism of injury into either guillotine (cut) or crush injury. Comorbid medical conditions included hypertension, diabetes, cardiovascular disease, and peripheral artery disease. Postoperative data collected included the anesthesia method, operating time, length of hospital stay, use of hyperbaric oxygen therapy (HBOT), the total number of HBOT sessions, and follow-up duration. All patients included in this study were followed for at least 6 months. Postoperative complications, including arterial insufficiency, infection, tip necrosis, and replantation failure, were defined as complications occurring after anastomosis. We compared the survival rates between those who were treated using the 2-point suture technique and those who were treated with the 3 or 4 sutures.

All study participants provided written informed consent for the storage of their medical information in the database and its use for research purposes. The study protocol was approved by the Institutional Review Board of the Kosin University Gospel Hospital of Korea (KUGH 2022-04-002). All procedures were performed in accordance with the ethical standards of the Institutional and National Research Committee and the 1964 Helsinki Declaration and its later amendments. This study was supported by a National Research Foundation of Korea (NRF) grant funded by the Korean government (MSIT) (No. 2020R1G1A1007678).

2.2. Statistical Analysis

A biomedical statistician analyzed the collected data. Statistical analysis was performed using SPSS version 27.0 (IBM Corp., Armonk, NY, USA). Patients' characteristics were summarized using means with SD or medians with interquartile ranges. Univariate analysis of patient characteristics and complications was conducted using a t-test and Kruskal-Wallis test for continuous variables, Pearson's chi-square test for categorical variables, and Fisher's exact test for variables with an expected frequency of less than 5. Odds ratios and 95% confidence intervals were obtained, and a p-value less than 0.05 was considered statistically significant.

2.3. Operative Procedure and Postoperative Management

Most of the replantations were performed under general anesthesia, and in some cases, nerve block and local anesthesia were performed. First, we found vessels that could be used in wounds and stumps, and vessel preparation for replantation followed standard techniques [14,15]. The 2-point suture technique for anastomosis was performed with 2-points at 180° intervals. A double arm 10-0 Nylon suture (Ethicon, Cornelia, Ga.) was used to pass the thread from the luminal side of the vessel to the outside of the vessel so that the margins were sufficiently everted. The same procedure was performed on the other side, after which a knot was made. Sutures were applied in the same way at the 180° point (Figure 1). We waited for reperfusion, and if blood leakage persisted, an additional suturing was performed in the leakage area. Anastomosis was performed by a senior author (H.-i.K.).

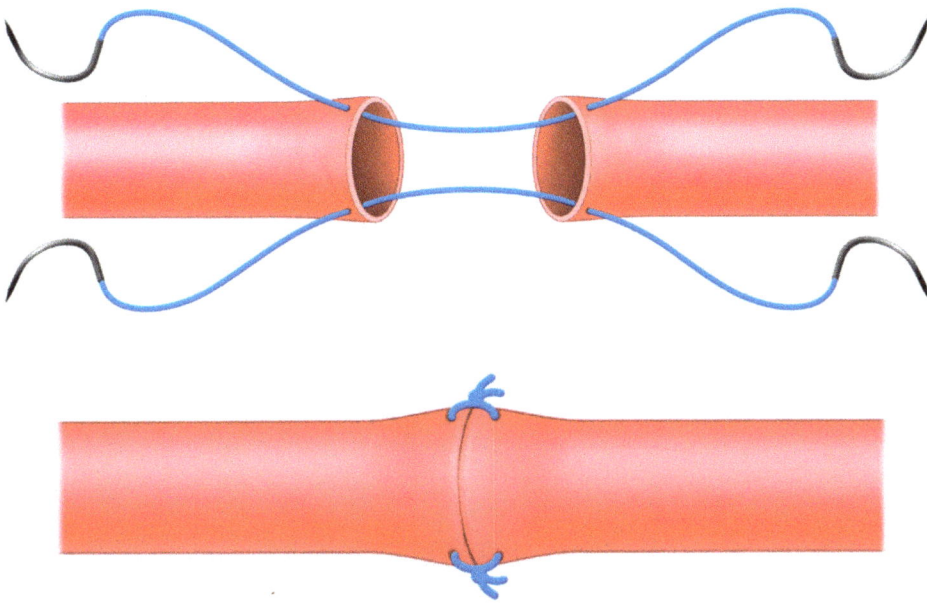

Figure 1. Schematic illustration of the 2-point suture technique.

In all the cases, close observation was followed by absolute bed rest for 3 days postoperatively. During monitoring, needle puncture exsanguination was performed if congestion occurred, and revision surgery was performed if arterial insufficiency occurred. If reperfusion was not achieved in the intraoperative field during revision surgery, a tie-over dressing was applied to the amputated part as a composite graft, and HBOT was performed to manage it in the form of a composite graft. By setting 2 atm and 100% oxygen in a hyperbaric chamber, HBOT was performed for 80 min every day for a week. The tie-over dressing for the composite graft was opened after 7 days. All patients were treated with 2 g of intravenous cefazedone sodium twice daily and prostaglandin E (alprostadil alpha-cyclodextrin). Survival was assessed on postoperative day 7, and the patient data, survival rates, and complications were reviewed.

3. Results

We enrolled 21 patients (thirteen male and eight female patients) who underwent replantation surgery with arterial anastomosis of vessels with a diameter of less than 0.3 mm between January 2017 and December 2021. The average age of the patients was 44.2 ± 15.1 years (range, 21–68 years). Among the patients, three had diabetes mellitus, three were active smokers, and one was a former smoker. The mechanisms of injury were crush (ten patients) and cut injuries (eleven patients). The injured lesions were on the forehead (one patient), thumb (two patients), index finger (six patients), middle finger (two patients), ring finger (four patients), small finger (five patients), and second toe (one patient). There were ten Tamai level I amputations and ten Tamai level II amputations [16]. In total, fifteen cases of replantation were performed under general anesthesia, three cases were performed under brachial plexus block, and the other three cases were performed under local anesthesia. The mean operating time was 145.2 ± 85.8 min (Table 1).

Table 1. Summarized patient and operative data *.

	Overall	2-Point Suture Group	3 or 4 Suture Group	p
No. of patients	21	12	9	
Survived	19 (90.5%)	11 (91.7%)	8 (88.9%)	1.0
Failed	2 (9.5%)	1 (8.3%)	1 (11.1%)	
Mean age, yrs	44.2 ± 15.1 (21–68)	43.6 ± 17.6 (21–68)	45.1 ± 10.8 (26–62)	0.83
Comorbidities				
Diabetes mellitus	3 (14.3%)	1 (8.3%)	2 (22.2%)	0.55
Active smoker	3 (14.3%)	2 (16.7%)	1 (11.1%)	1.0
Former smoker	1 (4.8%)	1 (8.3%)	0	1.0
Injury type				
Crush	9 (42.9%)	4 (33.3%)	5 (55.6%)	0.40
Cut	12 (57.1%)	8 (66.7%)	4 (44.4%)	0.40
Anesthesia method				
General	15 (71.4%)	9 (75%)	6 (66.7%)	1.0
Nerve block	3 (14.3%)	2 (16.7%)	1 (11.1%)	1.0
Local	3 (14.3%)	1 (8.3%)	2 (22.2%)	0.55
Mean operating time, min	145.2 ± 85.8 (50–360)	152.9 ± 82.4 (50–345)	135.0 ± 89.1 (50–360)	0.66
Replantation part				
Forehead	1 (4.8%)	0	1 (11.1%)	0.43
Finger	19 (90.5%)	12 (100%)	7 (77.8%)	0.17
Toe	1 (4.8%)	0	1 (11.1%)	0.43
Amputated level [†]				
Zone I	10 (47.6%)	6 (50%)	4 (44.4%)	1.0
Zone II	10 (47.6%)	6 (50%)	4 (44.4%)	1.0
No. Composite graft conversion and HBOT	9 (42.9%)	3 (25%)	6 (66.7%)	0.09
Mean hospital days	14.0 ± 4.4	13.8 ± 4.6	14.3 ± 4.1	0.78
Mean follow-up period, months	13.2 ± 1.8	13.1 ± 2.1	13.4 ± 1.2	0.67

* Values are expressed as median (interquartile range), n (%), mean ± SD, or mean (range). [†] Tamai classification for fingertip amputation.

Of the 21 replantation cases, 19 (90.5%) were successful. Further, the 2-point suture technique was performed in twelve cases, eleven of which survived. Three or four sutures were performed in nine cases, eight of whom survived. The two groups had no statistically significant differences with regard to age, sex, diabetes, or smoking history. Composite graft conversion was performed in three cases where the 2-point suture technique was used, and two of these cases survived. Composite graft conversion was performed in six cases where three or four sutures were used, five of which survived (Table 2). The survival rate was high in the cases where 2-point sutures were used (91.7% vs. 88.9%), and there were fewer cases of conversion to a composite graft (25.0% vs. 66.7%). However, the composite graft conversion rate and survival rate were not statistically significant according to the number of sutures. The average duration of hospital stay was 14.4 days (range: 5–21 days). The average follow-up duration was 13.2 months (range: 12–17 months).

Table 2. Patients' baseline characteristics and operative data.

Cases	Age (Years)/Sex	Mechanism of Injury	Injured Lesion	Anastomosis Stitches	Composite Graft and HBOT	Outcome
1	26/M	Crush	Forehead	3	X	Survived
2	52/F	Cut	LSF Zone I *	2	X	Survived
3	56/M	Crush	RSF Zone II *	4	O	Failed
4	49/M	Cut	RRF Zone II *	3	O	Survived

Table 2. Cont.

Cases	Age (Years)/Sex	Mechanism of Injury	Injured Lesion	Anastomosis Stitches	Composite Graft and HBOT	Outcome
5	21/M	Crush	RMF Zone I *	2	X	Survived
6	51/F	Crush	LRF Zone I *	3	O	Survived
7	65/M	Cut	LIF Zone II *	2	X	Survived
8	46/M	Cut	LIF Zone II *	3	X	Survived
9	26/F	Cut	LMF Zone II *	2	X	Survived
10	32/M	Crush	RT Zone II *	2	X	Survived
11	53/F	Cut	RT Zone I *	2	X	Survived
12	61/F	Cut	RIF Zone I *	2	O	Survived
13	45/M	Cut	RIF Zone I *	4	O	Survived
14	31/F	Cut	RSF Zone I *	4	O	Survived
15	21/M	Cut	RSF Zone II *	2	X	Survived
16	62/M	Crush	LSF Zone II *	3	O	Survived
17	68/M	Crush	RIF Zone I *	2	O	Survived
18	22/M	Cut	LRF Zone II *	2	X	Survived
19	42/M	Crush	RRF Zone II *	2	O	Failed
20	60/F	Cut	LIF Zone I *	2	X	Survived
21	40/F	Crush	L 2nd toe Zone I *	3	X	Survived

M, male; F, female; HBOT, hyperbaric oxygen therapy. RT, right thumb; RIF, right index finger; RMF, right middle finger; RRF, right ring finger; RSF, right small finger. LIF, left index finger; LMF, left middle finger; LRF, left ring finger; LSF, left small finger. * Tamai classification for fingertip amputation.

Two patients experienced arterial insufficiency. Wound exploration was performed immediately, and composite graft conversion was performed after re-anastomosis; however, replantation failed. After two weeks of dressing, surgical debridement and full-thickness skin grafting were performed.

- Case 1

A 60-year-old woman amputated her left index finger in a plant while using a fish-cutting machine. One digital pulp artery could be found at the site of amputation after debridement of the stump tissue and was anastomosed using the 2-point suture technique. The fingertip survived successfully, and three months postoperatively, the patient did not have any complications or functional impairment (Figure 2).

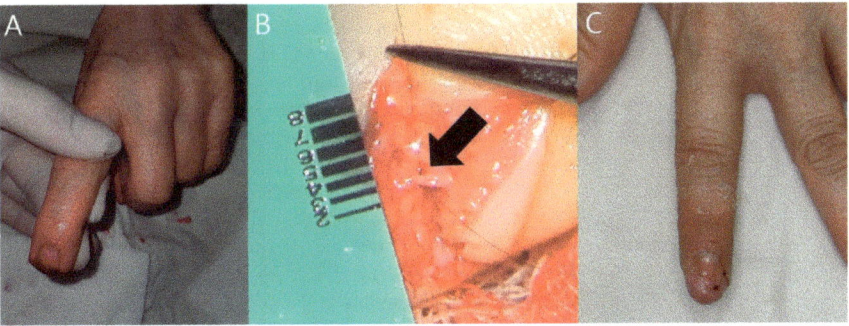

Figure 2. Case 1 (patient 20). (**A**) A 60-year-old patient with an amputated left index finger. (**B**) Black arrow indicates the vessel that was anastomosed using the 2-point suture technique. (**C**) Three months postoperatively, the patient did not complain of any functional complications.

- Case 2

A 61-year-old woman amputated her right index finger in a plant while using an abalone-cutting machine. One digital pulp artery could be found at the site of amputation after debridement of the stump tissue and was anastomosed using the 2-point suture technique. However, the color of the flap became pale in the evening, and arterial insufficiency was noted, so a wound re-exploration was performed, but reperfusion was not achieved. Composite graft conversion was performed after arteriorrhaphy, and it was confirmed that the graft was engrafted seven days after surgery. The fingertip survived successfully, and nine months postoperatively, the patient did not have any complications or functional impairment (Figure 3).

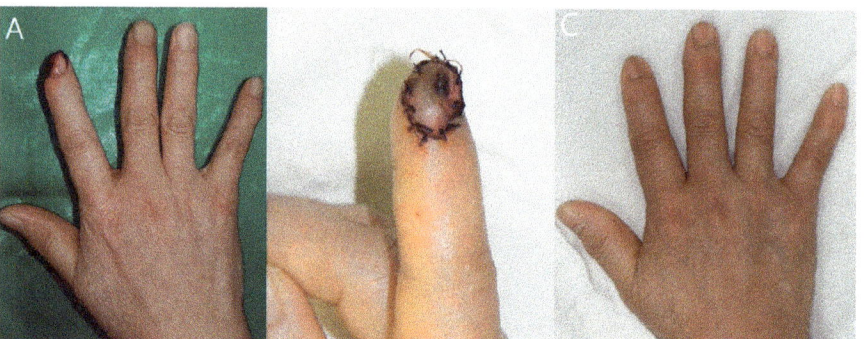

Figure 3. Case 2 (patient 12). (**A**) A 61-year-old patient with an amputated right index finger. (**B**) The tie-over dressing was removed on postoperative day 7. The stump was well maintained. (**C**) Nine months postoperatively, the patient did not complain of any functional complications.

4. Discussion

This review suggests that the 2-point suture technique is relatively safe and feasible for microvascular anastomosis. In this study, survival rates were compared between cases where the 2-point suture technique was used and cases where three or four sutures were used. In the 2-point suture group, 11 out of 12 cases survived, and the composite graft conversion rate was 25.0%. In contrast, eight out of nine cases in which three or four sutures were used survived, and the conversion rate was 66.7%. Hence, the outcomes of the 2-point suture technique were satisfactory. We thought that cases with three or four sutures could have poor outcomes due to occlusion of the lumen by the thickness of the suture material and the number of sutures.

The first microscopic surgery was performed in 1921 by Carl Nylen, an otolaryngologist in Stockholm, Sweden [17]. In 1960, Jacobson used a microscope for the first time in vascular surgery for carotid anastomosis in dogs [18]. Since then, further development has continued, and improvements in microsurgical tools, suture materials, vascular clamps, and microscopes have made supermicrosurgery possible [19–21]. Koshima et al. published the first use of a perforator flap, the deep inferior epigastric skin flap, in 1989, which heralded the development of a variety of different perforator flaps in the following years [22]. Koshima reported the first use of flaps based on perforator vessels with a caliber of less than 0.8 mm at the First International Course on Perforator Flap and Arterialized Skin Flaps in 1997. The ability to use such small vessels for anastomosis was significant because it greatly increased the surgeon's freedom in selecting free tissue flaps while at the same time reducing donor site morbidity by preserving fascia, muscles, nerves, and major vessels during the dissection. Koshima et al. first called this technique "supramicrosurgery" in their description of the paraumbilical perforator flap in 1998 [23]. In 2007, Koshima again referred to the technique as "supermicrosurgery" at the first international meeting on innovative microsurgical technology and published a definition of the procedure in 2010 [24]. A consensus on the name "supermicrosurgery" was reached at the First European Conference on Supermicrosurgery held in Barcelona in March 2010 [25]. Supermicrosurgery has many advantages, but its biggest advantage is that it can reduce surgical time and donor site morbidity [25]. Supermicrosurgery is the latest trend in reconstructive surgery and has enabled new flap designs and free tissue transfers, as well as lymphovenous anastomosis [24,25]. However, supermicrosurgery requires considerable technique, as well as specialized instruments and microscopes [25]. In particular, supermicrosurgery requires a higher skill level of eye–microscope–hand coordination, more dexterous tissue handling, and more refined motor skills than microsurgery [26]. A number of training methods have been developed to teach these skills. Among these, the Chen et al. chicken thigh model allows trainees to learn the skills in a comfortable way and to become familiar with the instrument [26]. In the chicken thigh model, the branch of the ischiatic artery and vein is 0.3–0.5 mm, which is optimized for supermicrosurgical practice [26].

Various suture techniques have also been developed, including the simple interrupted microvascular suture, the 12 o'clock to 6 o'clock method, the 3 o'clock to 9 o'clock-side-side method, the triangulation method, and the posterior wall first [1,4,27]. The first description of the 12 o'clock to 6 o'clock microvascular surgery technique is difficult to find in the literature. This technique is considered to be the most basic and is most often referred to as the conventional method of performing a simple interrupted microvascular anastomosis [28]. In this method, the first suture is placed at 12 o'clock (also sometimes referred to as 0 degrees), and the second stitch is placed at 6 o'clock (or 180 degrees). The third and fourth sutures are placed at 2 o'clock and 4 o'clock to complete the anterior wall. The vessel is then turned over 180 degrees with a clamp, and the fifth and sixth sutures are placed at 8 o'clock and 10 o'clock [28]. The main disadvantage of this technique is the need to rotate the vessel 180 degrees to suture the posterior wall, which can potentially cause blood vessel damage. In 1986, Yu et al. presented a method to perform the first suture on the posterior wall and the second suture at a 90 degree angle to the anterior wall to facilitate the remaining sutures and named it the 3 o'clock to 9 o'clock-side-side method [29]. Perform the third, fourth, and fifth sutures on the anterior wall, turn 90 degrees, and perform the remaining three sutures on the posterior wall. According to the authors, the 90-degree rotation reduces potential damage to the endothelium compared to the traditional 180-degree rotation and is easier than suturing the posterior wall first [29]. The triangulation method was first developed by Alexis Carrel in 1902 [30]. It is a method in which three standard stitches are made at an angle of 120 degrees, and then two more stitches are made between each stitch. The lumen can be lifted with two standard stitches, reducing the number of cases where the posterior wall is sutured together [30]. The posterior wall first technique was first described by Harris et al. in 1981 [31]. This technique is also sometimes called the "backup" technique. The first suture is placed in the center of the posterior wall, with the second and third sutures placed on either side of the first. The fourth and fifth sutures are placed adjacent to the second and third, advancing anteriorly on either side, leaving a long tail to facilitate the placement of the sixth and seventh sutures. Similarly, both the sixth and seventh sutures are left long to facilitate the placement of the last suture, which is placed equidistant from the sixth and the seventh. Advantages include constant visualization of the back wall, which reduces the risk of accidentally catching the back wall. Harris et al. concluded that the posterior wall first technique is less complicated, faster, and easier to perform than the anterior wall technique [31].

Amputation is one of the most common cases in emergency departments. Particularly in the case of distal fingertip amputations, microsurgical vascular anastomosis may not be possible, and composite grafts are often used in such nonreplantable fingertip amputations [32]. However, some studies have shown that these composite grafts have good results in treating pediatric fingertip amputations but have a low success rate in adults [33,34]. To increase the success rate of composite grafts in adults, Chen et al. chose to increase the contact area and reduce unnecessary graft thickness [32]. Excision of the bone fragment and defatting of the pulp fat pad on the distal amputated fingertip reduced the thickness of the graft. Circumferential deepithelialization of the amputated stump provided maximum contact surface between the distal amputated fingertip and the wound base. Tie-over wet gauze dressing and finger splinting immobilized the injured fingertip and minimized the risk of a postoperative wound base hematoma and incidental detachment of the graft.

These procedures helped adult patients achieve an overall graft survival rate of 93.5% for fingertip amputation [32]. The authors also used the above method when graft conversion was required, according to this study. There were nine cases of graft conversion, seven of which were successful. Composite grafts can be a good alternative for nonreplantable fingertip amputations.

HBOT is a treatment modality in which the patient inhales 100% O_2 at high atmospheric pressure, and it is well known to have a positive effect on wound healing [35]. Systemic HBOT increases oxygen diffusion in the vessels to improve the condition of ischemia-reperfusion injuries and stimulate angiogenesis [35]. HBOT in plastic surgery is used for wounds, burns, crush injuries, infection, and flap surgery. Previous animal studies have shown that the application of HBOT to composite grafts in rats and rabbits increases graft survival [36,37]. Fordor et al. used 20 Sprague-Dawley rats to harvest 3×3 cm skin from the back, sutured the skin to the fascia, and performed a composite graft. Further, by setting 202 kPa and 100% oxygen in a hyperbaric chamber, HBOT was performed for 90 min every day for 2 weeks, and the survival area was larger than that of the control group [36]. Li et al. conducted a rabbit experiment using an auricular composite graft, which is useful for skin defects [37]. They used 24 New Zealand White rabbits to harvest 5 mm, 1 cm, and 2 cm sized circular chondrocutaneous composite grafts from the auricle, and the grafts were sutured to the back. Moreover, by setting 2.4 atm and 100% oxygen in a hyperbaric chamber, HBOT was performed for 90 min, a total of 7 times in 5 days, and the graft survival rate was higher than that of the control group in larger composite grafts [37]. Lee et al. reported that HBOT increased the composite graft survival rate and shortened the graft-healing period in patients with fingertip amputation [38]. HBOT includes intermittent administration of 100% oxygen at pressures >1 atm in a pressure vessel [38]. The arterial PO_2 increased to 1000–1500 mmHg owing to dissolved oxygen in the plasma. At tissue and cellular levels, hyperoxygenation promotes angiogenesis and improves post-ischemic tissue survival. Increasing the applied pressure increases the PO_2 of tissues, which is beneficial for wound healing [39,40]. The authors performed composite graft conversion in cases of replantation failure and applied 2 atm HBOT for 80 min for a week. All patients tolerated it well and achieved good results.

A limitation of this study was the small sample size and the use of Nylon 10-0 sutures. Due to the small sample size, influencing factors such as age, comorbidities, level of injury, and mechanism of injury may not have been properly assessed. However, the authors' study did not show a statistically significant difference, and when more samples are collected, the factors associated with the prognosis of anastomosed vessels will be studied. Sutures can also act as foreign bodies or obstacles; therefore, if thinner threads (Nylon 11-0 or smaller sutures) were used, the outcomes of using three or four sutures may have improved [4]. Nowadays, with supermicrosurgical tools, the authors also use 11-0 Nylon, a superfine tip forceps, and perform a lymphovenous anastomosis. In this situation, four to six sutures are performed. Even in the case of microvascular anastomosis at the proximal site, sutures are performed as much as possible to maintain the lumen. However, this technique is an option that can be used in an emergency situation when proper instruments are not available. This study has confirmed that better results can be achieved by attempting the 2-point suture technique rather than many sutures or abandoning vascular sutures due to lack of an instrument.

5. Conclusions

The results of this study suggest that the 2-point suture technique is a feasible alternative to placing three or four sutures in microvascular anastomosis. This option may be useful in situations where supermicrosurgical tools are not available. Composite graft conversion and HBOT can be the second choice for reconstruction when replantation failure is suspected.

Author Contributions: Conceptualization, B.-s.K. and H.-i.K.; methodology, J.-h.P.; formal analysis, H.-s.Y.; investigation, B.-s.K., H.-s.Y., and H.-i.K.; resources, H.-s.Y. and H.-i.K.; data curation, B.-s.K. and Y.-s.K.; writing—original draft preparation, B.-s.K. and H.-i.K.; writing—review and editing, H.-s.Y. and H.-i.K.; visualization, J.-h.P.; supervision, J.-h.P. and Y.-s.K. All authors have read and agreed to the published version of the manuscript.

Funding: This study was supported by a National Research Foundation of Korea grant funded by the Korean government Ministry of Science and ICT (No. 2020R1G1A1007678).

Institutional Review Board Statement: The study was conducted in accordance with the Declaration of Helsinki and approved by the Institutional Review Board of Kosin University Gospel Hospital of Korea (KUGH-IRB 2022-04-002; date of approval, 12 April 2022).

Informed Consent Statement: Informed consent was obtained from all subjects involved in the study.

Data Availability Statement: Not applicable.

Conflicts of Interest: The authors declare no conflict of interest. The funders had no role in the design of the study; in the collection, analyses, or interpretation of data; in the writing of the manuscript; or in the decision to publish the results.

References

1. Alghoul, M.S.; Gordon, C.R.; Yetman, R.; Buncke, G.M.; Siemionow, M.; Afifi, A.M.; Moon, W.K. From simple interrupted to complex spiral: A systematic review of various suture techniques for microvascular anastomoses. *Microsurgery* **2011**, *31*, 72–80. [CrossRef] [PubMed]
2. Mofikoya, B.O.; Ugburo, A.O.; Bankole, O.B. Microvascular anastomosis of Vessels less than 0.5 mm in Diameter: A Supermicrosurgery Training Model in Lagos, Nigeria. *J. Hand Microsurg.* **2011**, *3*, 15–17. [CrossRef] [PubMed]
3. Huang, C.D.; Chow, S.P.; Chan, C.W. Experience with anastomoses of arteries approximately 0.20 mm in external diameter. *Plast. Reconstr. Surg.* **1982**, *69*, 299–305. [CrossRef] [PubMed]
4. Turan, T.; Ozçelik, D.; Kuran, I.; Sadikoglu, B.; Bas, L.; San, T.; Sungun, A. Eversion with four sutures: An easy, fast, and reliable technique for microvascular anastomosis. *Plast. Reconstr. Surg.* **2001**, *107*, 463–470. [CrossRef] [PubMed]
5. Akentieva, T.N.; Ovcharenko, E.A.; Kudryavtseva, Y.A. Influence of suture material on the development of postoperative complications in vascular surgery and their prevention. *Khirurgiia* **2019**, *10*, 75–81. [CrossRef]
6. Dahlke, H.; Dociu, N.; Thurau, K. Thrombogenicity of different suture materials as revealed by scanning electron microscopy. *J. Biomed. Mater. Res.* **1980**, *14*, 251–268. [CrossRef]
7. Ozkan, O.; Ozgentaş, H.E. Open guide suture technique for safe microvascular anastomosis. *Ann. Plast. Surg.* **2005**, *55*, 289–291.
8. Miyamoto, S.; Sakuraba, M.; Asano, T.; Tsuchiya, S.; Hamamoto, Y.; Onoda, S.; Tomori, Y.; Yasunaga, Y.; Harii, K. Optimal technique for microvascular anastomosis of very small vessels: Comparative study of three techniques in a rat superficial inferior epigastric arterial flap model. *J. Plast. Reconstr. Aesthet. Surg.* **2010**, *63*, 1196–1201. [CrossRef]
9. Cobbett, J. Small vessel anastomosis. A comparison of suture techniques. *Br. J. Plast. Surg.* **1967**, *20*, 16–20. [CrossRef]
10. Harashina, T. Use of the united suture in microvascular anastomoses. *Plast. Reconstr. Surg* **1977**, *59*, 134–135. [CrossRef]
11. Harashina, T.; Irigaray, A. Expansion of smaller vessel diameter by fish-mouth incision in microvascular anastomosis with marked size discrepancy. *Plast. Reconstr. Surg.* **1980**, *65*, 502–503. [CrossRef]
12. Foo, T.L. Open guide suture technique for distal fingertip replantation. *J. Plast. Reconstr. Aesthet. Surg.* **2013**, *66*, 443–444. [CrossRef]
13. Cifuentes, I.J.; Rodriguez, J.R.; Yanes, R.A.; Salisbury, M.C.; Cuadra, Á.J.; Varas, J.E.; Dagnino, B.L. A Novel Ex Vivo Training Model for Acquiring Supermicrosurgical Skills Using a Chicken Leg. *J. Reconstr. Microsug.* **2016**, *32*, 699–705. [CrossRef]
14. Kim, J.S.; Yang, J.W.; Lee, D.C.; Ki, S.H.; Roh, S.Y. Challenges in fingertip replantation. *Semin. Plast. Surg.* **2013**, *27*, 165–173.
15. Hattori, Y.; Doi, K.; Sakamoto, S.; Yamasaki, H.; Wahegaonkar, A.; Addosooki, A. Fingertip replantation. *J. Hand Surg. Am.* **2007**, *32*, 548–555. [CrossRef]
16. Tamai, S. Twenty years' experience of limb replantation—Review of 293 upper extremity replants. *J. Hand Surg. Am.* **1982**, *7*, 549–556. [CrossRef]
17. Nylen, C.O. The Microscope in Aural Surgery, Its First Use and Later Development. *Acta Otolaryngol. Suppl.* **1954**, *116*, 226–240. [CrossRef]
18. Jacobson, J.H., II; Suarez, E.L. Microsurgery in anastomosis of small vessels. *Surg. Forum* **1960**, *11*, 243–245.
19. Jacobson, J.H., II. Founder's lecture in plastic surgery. *Ann. Plast. Surg.* **2006**, *56*, 471–474. [CrossRef]
20. Jacobson, J.H., II. The early days of microsurgery in Vermont. *Mt. Sinai J. Med.* **1997**, *64*, 160–163.
21. Acland, R. New instruments for microvascular surgery. *Br. J. Surg.* **1972**, *59*, 181–184. [CrossRef] [PubMed]
22. Koshima, I.; Soeda, S. Inferior epigastric artery skin flaps without rectus abdominis muscle. *Br. J. Plast. Surg.* **1989**, *42*, 645–648. [CrossRef] [PubMed]

23. Koshima, I.; Inagawa, K.; Urushibara, K.; Moriguchi, T. Paraumbilical perforator flap without deep inferior epigastric vessels. *Plast. Reconstr. Surg.* **1998**, *102*, 1052–1057. [CrossRef] [PubMed]
24. Koshima, I.; Yamamoto, T.; Narushima, M.; Mihara, M.; Iida, T. Perforator flaps and supermicrosurgery. *Clin. Plast. Surg.* **2010**, *37*, 683–689. [CrossRef]
25. Masia, J.; Olivares, L.; Koshima, I.; Teo, T.C.; Suominen, S.; Van Landuyt, K.; Demirtas, Y.; Becker, C.; Pons, G.; Garusi, C.; et al. Barcelona consensus on supermicrosurgery. *J. Reconstr. Microsurg.* **2014**, *30*, 53–58. [CrossRef]
26. Chen, W.F.; Eid, A.; Yamamoto, T.; Keith, J.; Nimmons, G.L.; Lawrence, W.T. A novel supermicrosurgery training model: The chicken thigh. *J. Plast. Reconstr. Aesthet. Surg.* **2014**, *67*, 973–978. [CrossRef]
27. Firsching, R.; Terhaag, P.D.; Müller, W.; Frowein, R.A. Continuous and interrupted suture technique in microsurgical end-to-end anastomosis. *Microsurgery* **1984**, *5*, 80–84. [CrossRef]
28. Hou, S.M.; Seaber, A.V.; Urbaniak, J.R. An alternative technique of microvascular anastomosis. *Microsurgery* **1987**, *8*, 22–24. [CrossRef]
29. Yu, H.L.; Sagi, A.; Ferder, M.; Strauch, B. A simplified technique for endto-end microanastomosis. *J. Reconstr. Microsurg.* **1986**, *2*, 191–194. [CrossRef]
30. Kim, E.; Singh, M.; Akelina, Y.; Shurey, S.; Myers, S.R.; Ghanem, A.M. Effect of microvascular anastomosis technique on end product outcome in simulated training: A prospective blinded randomized controlled trial. *J. Reconstr. Microsurg.* **2016**, *32*, 556–561. [CrossRef]
31. Harris, G.D.; Finseth, F.; Buncke, H.J. Posterior-wall-first microvascular anastomotic technique. *Br. J. Plast. Surg.* **1981**, *34*, 47–49. [CrossRef]
32. Chen, S.Y.; Wang, C.H.; Fu, J.P.; Chang, S.C.; Chen, S.G. Composite grafting for traumatic fingertip amputation in adults: Technique reinforcement and experience in 31 digits. *J. Trauma* **2011**, *70*, 148–153. [CrossRef]
33. Moiemen, N.S.; Elliot, D. Composite graft replacement of digital tips. 2. A study in children. *J. Hand Surg. Br.* **1997**, *22*, 346–352. [CrossRef]
34. Uysal, A.; Kankaya, Y.; Ulusoy, M.G.; Sungur, N.; Karalezli, N.; Kayran, O.; Koçer, U. An alternative technique for microsurgically unreplantable fingertip amputations. *Ann. Plast. Surg.* **2006**, *57*, 545–551. [CrossRef]
35. Thom, S.R. Hyperbaric oxygen: Its mechanisms and efficacy. *Plast. Reconstr. Surg.* **2011**, *127*, 131S–141S. [CrossRef]
36. Fodor, L.; Ramon, Y.; Meilik, B.; Carmi, N.; Shoshani, O.; Ullmann, Y. Effect of hyperbaric oxygen on survival of composite grafts in rats. *Scand. J. Plast. Reconstr. Surg. Hand Surg.* **2006**, *40*, 257–260. [CrossRef]
37. Li, E.N.; Menon, N.G.; Rodriguez, E.D.; Norkunas, M.; Rosenthal, R.E.; Goldberg, N.H.; Silverman, R.P. The effect of hyperbaric oxygen therapy on composite graft survival. *Ann. Plast. Surg.* **2004**, *53*, 141–145. [CrossRef]
38. Lee, Y.S.; Heo, J.W.; Moon, J.S.; Kim, S.W.; Kim, J.Y. Effects of hyperbaric oxygen on graft survival outcomes in composite grafting for amputated fingertip injury. *Arch. Plast. Surg.* **2020**, *47*, 444–450. [CrossRef]
39. Eskes, A.; Vermeulen, H.; Lucas, C.; Ubbink, D.T. Hyperbaric oxygen therapy for treating acute surgical and traumatic wounds. *Cochrane Database Syst. Rev.* **2013**, *16*, CD008059. [CrossRef]
40. Dauwe, P.B.; Pulikkottil, B.J.; Lavery, L.; Stuzin, J.M.; Rohrich, R.J. Does hyperbaric oxygen therapy work in facilitating acute wound healing: A systematic review. *Plast. Reconstr. Surg.* **2014**, *133*, 208e–215e. [CrossRef]

Disclaimer/Publisher's Note: The statements, opinions and data contained in all publications are solely those of the individual author(s) and contributor(s) and not of MDPI and/or the editor(s). MDPI and/or the editor(s) disclaim responsibility for any injury to people or property resulting from any ideas, methods, instructions or products referred to in the content.

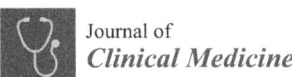

Article

Use of a Fibula Free Flap for Mandibular Reconstruction in Severe Craniofacial Microsomia in Children with Obstructive Sleep Apnea

Krzysztof Dowgierd [1,*], Rafał Pokrowiecki [2], Andrzej Myśliwiec [3] and Łukasz Krakowczyk [4]

1 Department of Clinical Pediatrics, Head and Neck Surgery Clinic for Children and Young Adults, University of Warmia and Mazury, Żołnierska 18a Street, 10-561 Olsztyn, Poland
2 Craniofacial Center, Regional Specialized Children's Hospital in Olsztyn, 10-561 Olsztyn, Poland
3 Institute of Physiotherapy and Health Science, The Jerzy Kukuczka Academy of Physical Education in Katowice, Ul. Mikołowska 72A, 40-065 Katowice, Poland
4 Oncological and Reconstructive Surgery Clinic, Branch of National Oncological Institute in Gliwice, Maria Sklodowska-Curie Institute—Oncology Centre (MSCI), Ul. Wybrzeże Armii Krajowej 15, 44-100 Gliwice, Poland
* Correspondence: krzysztofdowgierd@gmail.com

Abstract: This is a retrospective study describing a multi-stage protocol for the management of severe mandibular hypoplasia in craniofacial microsomia (CFM) with accompanying obstructive sleep apnea (OSA). Patients with severe mandibular hypoplasia require reconstruction functionality and esthetical features. In the cohort, reconstructions based on free fibular flaps (FFF) may be the most effective way. Patients aged 4–17 years with severe mandibular hypoplasia were treated with FFF, which initially improved the respiratory function assessed on polysomnography (AHI). In the next stages of treatment of cases with respiratory deterioration, it was indicated to perform distraction osteogenesis (DO) of the mandible and the structures reconstructed with FFF. All surgeries were planned in accordance with virtual surgery planning VSP. The aim of the study was to prospectively assess the effectiveness of multi-stage mandibular reconstruction in craniofacial microsomia with the use of a free fibula flap in terms of improving respiratory failure due to obstructive sleep apnea (OSA). The FFF reconstruction method, performed with virtual surgical planning (VSP), is proving to be an effective alternative to traditional methods of mandibular reconstruction in patients with severe CFM with OSA.

Keywords: craniofacial microsomia; obstructive sleep apnea; free fibular flaps; microsurgical reconstruction

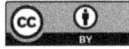

1. Introduction

The aim of the study was to retrospective assess the effectiveness of multi-stage mandibular reconstruction in craniofacial microsomia (CMF) with the use of a free fibula flap (FFF) in terms of improving respiratory failure due to OSA.

Craniofacial microsomia is the second most common congenital disorder of the head and neck. The occurrence of its severe form is rare. Mandibular hypoplasia is a feature of CFM. Other abnormalities include facial nerve palsy, ear anomalies, or facial soft tissue deficit on the same side [1]. The mandible is often the most functionally affected structure [2–4].

A possible treatment for mandibular hypoplasia in neonates and infants is mandibular distraction, but this is not possible when a mandibular bone is missing [5,6]. It becomes necessary to perform mandibular reconstruction, which enables further DO. Mandibular deficiencies can be corrected by bone grafting, distraction osteogenesis, or a combination of these methods [7]. In the case of patients with severe craniofacial microsomia, satisfactory correction is difficult to achieve with traditional methods. Most cases of CFM are well managed by conventional techniques, including costochondral grafts (CCG). Mandibular reconstruction is beneficial in CFM to address functional problems, such as airway and facial symmetry, mandibular and maxillary growth, and dental development. The application of conventional techniques may be limited in cases with severe mandibular displacement.

Free fibular flap reconstruction (FFFR) has been introduced as a new treatment option for patients with severe CFM. For patients with severe mandibular hypoplasia, FFFR may prove to be the most effective way of restoring mandibular shape and function [8]. The use of free tissue transfer for head and neck reconstruction has been proven to be safe and effective in the pediatric population [9–11].

The term obstructive sleep apnea (OSA) describes a syndrome of upper airway dysfunction during sleep that is characterized by increased upper airway resistance and the collapse of the throat. Symptoms of sleep apnea include snoring and/or increased work of breathing during sleep. Obstructive apnea includes many clinical entities of varying severities. It is characterized by snoring, labored breathing during sleep, and periods of complete or partial obstruction. Because OSA is associated with neurodevelopmental, metabolic, and cardiovascular consequences, an accurate diagnosis based on a patient examination and polysomnography (PSG) is important. Studies on the prevalence of OSA in patients with CFM have shown high variability, ranging from 7% to 67%. According to the authors, patients with severe face deformities are at risk for severe forms of OSA [12,13]. Children with various craniofacial conditions have been shown to be at increased risk for upper airway obstruction. The lack of prospective studies makes the prevalence of OSA and the causes of OSA in this population difficult to determine. OSA is the result of both structural factors that reduce airway size and neuromotor deficits that impair the patient's ability to maintain an open airway during sleep. Structural factors, such as a retracted and underdeveloped mandible, cause a reduction in the volume of the upper airway by shifting all structures backwards, closing the volume of the upper airway. Craniofacial diseases cause the dysfunction of the muscles of the mouth and throat, which affects swallowing, speech, and breathing. In children with craniofacial deformity, the ratio of length to tension of the muscles of the upper respiratory tract is changed, preventing them from working efficiently. One of the most common impairments in children with craniofacial disorders is feeding. This usually results in longer feeding times and can cause other problems, including malnutrition, dehydration, or aspiration of contents into the upper respiratory tract. Infants with craniofacial defects are at risk of poor growth, especially early in life. Sudden death during sleep may also occur in this group. Other symptoms of OSA in children include difficulty breathing while sleeping, drowsiness and night awakenings, learning disabilities, neurocognitive deficits, or failure to thrive. Obstructive sleep apnea is a serious disorder that manifests itself in excessive sleepiness. OSA is an independent risk factor for hypertension, ischemic heart disease, stroke, heart failure, atrial fibrillation, insulin resistance, and sudden death [14,15].

2. Materials and Methods

The records of patients who presented with severe CFM with mandible hypoplasia classified as severe, according to Pruzansky III, and who were treated were reviewed retrospectively (Table 1).

The inclusion criteria were related to the treatment protocol used at our department, for confirmed CFM with severe mandibular hypoplasia and the deterioration of OSA, as confirmed on examination and PSG (AHI). The treatment indications included deteriorating respiratory disorders confirmed by clinical symptoms and PSG. The factors qualifying for the primary reconstruction were severe mandible defect and worsening clinical symptoms and sleep parameters in PSG. The conservative definition of pediatric OSA [16] is AHI < 1 = normal, AHI 1–5.0 = mild, AHI 5.1–9.9 = moderate, and AHI > 10 = severe. The factors qualifying for mandibular distraction in the next stage included deteriorating clinical parameters and AHI on PSG [17].

Table 1. Characteristics of patients with HFM based on age, gender, side of deformity, determination of mandibular deformity based on Pruzansky classification, and determination of additional facial and general developmental deformities.

Age at 1st Operation y.o.	Gender	Side	Pruzansky	Additional Deformations of Face	Other Deformations
4	Female	Left	III	Soft tissue atrophy	
4	Male	Left	III	Microtia, atresia, VII palsy, soft tissue atrophy	
4	Female	Left	III	Microtia, atresia, VII palsy, soft tissue atrophy, orbital dystopia, cervical spinal deformation	
5	Male	Left	III	Cleft LP orbital dystopia anoftalmia, mictai, VII palsy, soft tissue atrophy	Cervical spinal deformation, scoliosis
5	Female	Right	III	Microtia, atresia, VII palsy, soft tissue atrophy	
5	Male	Left	IIB	Microtia, atresia, VII palsy, soft tissue atrophy	Forearm deformation, cervical spinal deformation
5	Female	Right	IIB	Microtia, atresia, VII palsy, soft tissue atrophy	Forearm deformation
7	Male	Right	III	Microtia, atresia, VII palsy, soft tissue atrophy, orbital dystopia, deformation Cleft Tessier 11/4	Cervical spinal deformation
8	Male	Left	III	Microtia, atresia, VII palsy, soft tissue atrophy, orbital dystopia, cervical spinal deformation	
9	Male	Left	IIB	Microtia, atresia, VII palsy, soft tissue atrophy	
14	Male	Right	IIB	Microtia, atresia, VII palsy, soft tissue atrophy	
15	Female	Right	Bilat III/II B	Microtia, atresia, soft tissue atrophy	
17	Male	Right	III	Microtia, atresia, VII palsy, soft tissue atrophy	

The exclusion criteria included the absence of signed informed consent; a low body mass index; general health problems; no respiratory distress and central respiratory distress; disqualification for an anesthetic reason; disqualification for ENT reasons, such as tracheomalacia, laryngomalacia, or tonsil hyperplasia; and irregular or no reporting to requested follow-ups or the final follow-up.

The assessment of AHI was the basis for the qualification for surgery and evaluation of the surgery outcome. Patients who presented a decrease in AHI on follow-up PSG after mandibular FFFR required subsequent mandible DO.

Teenage patients were qualified for bimaxillary surgery, temporomandibular joint prosthesis, or both.

Patients qualified for mandibular FFFR underwent pre-operative planning. Surgical templates were prepared for bone cutting of both the mandibular defect and osteotomy of the fibula, as well as production stereolithographic models. Virtual planning and individual implants were used in accordance with manufacturer recommendations (CHM, Poland, Stare Juchy). The surgery involved FFF harvesting and FFF modifications, including the selection of the donor fibula, the site and the type of neck vessels used for anastomosis, the location of a skin island, and the preparation of segmental osteotomies of fibula, applied individually to each case.

A CT scan was performed before the surgery to prepare for virtual planning. Then a CT was carried out after the surgery to control and assess the correctness of the performed reconstruction. In the protocol, follow-up CT scans were performed 6 months after the surgery, before the removal of the stabilizing plates. No imaging examinations were performed in the following years. The next examination was performed just before the mandibular DO to assess the amount of bone and to plan the position of the distance device and the osteotomy line.

3. Results

The treatment of 13 patients with severe craniofacial microsomia was analyzed retrospectively.

Among the 13 patients, three started treatments at the age of 4, four at the age of 5, and then at the age of 7, 8, 9, 14, and 15 years, one patient at each age. The study group included five girls and eight boys. The patients' follow-up period ranged from 15 to 77 months (mean 39.00). In seven patients, the mandible was deformed on the left side, and in the other six, on the right side. Before treatment, two patients underwent unsuccessful treatment attempts in other centers: these were free CCG. The first patient was 5 years old, and the other was 7 years old.

All patients underwent the reconstruction of the ramus and body of the mandible deficit with FFF microvascular flaps. In four patients, one fibular fragment was used, and in the other nine patients, two bone fragments of FFF were used. In four patients, no skin island was used, and in the remaining nine, a skin island was used to correct the deficit of soft tissues (Table 2; Figures 1 and 2).

In the patients who additionally had a soft tissue flap, only two had a single-element bone fragment. In four patients, an additional unilateral sagittal split osteotomy was performed on the opposite side. These were patients in whom a two-component FFF was used to reconstruct the mandibular ramus and body. Two patients developed complications in the partial resorption of the bone graft, and in one patient, despite the healing of the skin island, complete resorption of the bone part of the graft occurred. Virtual planning with templates and individual implants was only not used in two patients. They were treated with single element FFF grafts.

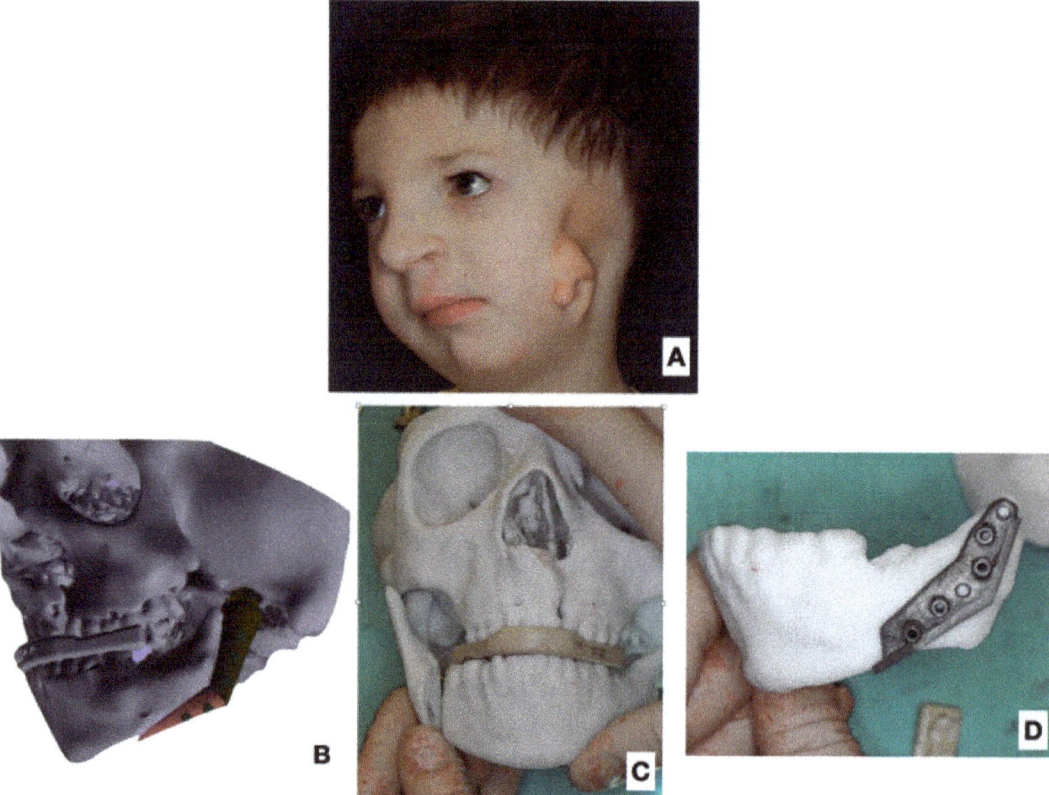

Figure 1. Patient 5 years old with HF Pruzansky III. (**A**) Three-quarter view, soft tissue deformity visible, with auricle microtia. (**B**) 3D image reconstruction with planned free fibular flap reconstruction. (**C**) Stereolithographic model for intraoperative planning and control. (**D**) Stereolithographic model with intraoperative template.

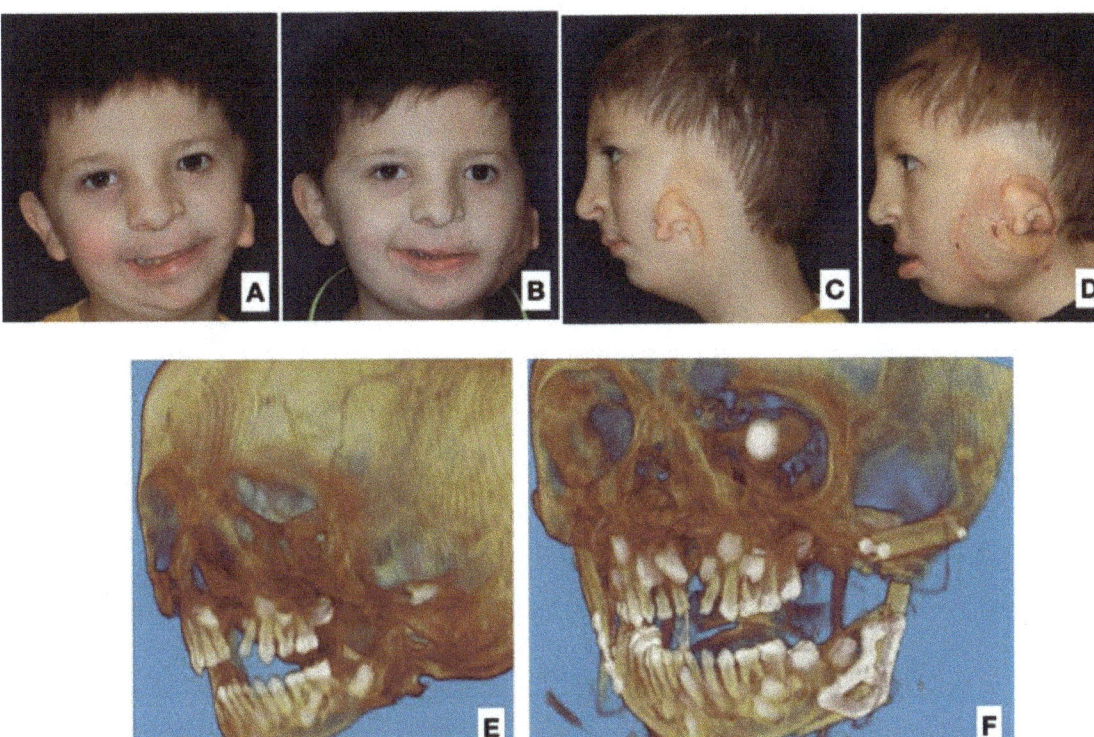

Figure 2. (**A**) Frontal view before surgery, showing asymmetry and soft tissue deficit. (**B**) View one month after surgery with visible correction of asymmetry and soft tissue deficit. (**C**) Side view before surgery. (**D**) Side view one month after surgery, visible insertion in cheek area. (**E**) Preoperative 3D image reconstruction. (**F**) 3D image reconstruction after surgery and mandibular FFF reconstruction.

Table 2. Characteristics of free flaps used for mandibular reconstruction in patients with HFM with definition of the affected side, number of bony elements of the fibular flap, collection of the skin island, reconstruction of the mandibular anatomical region, use of additional osteotomies during mandibular reconstruction with a free flap based on microvascular anastomoses, occurrence of complications during and after surgery, use of virtual planning and individual implants (VSP, IPS), follow-up period after reconstruction. CCG—costochondral graft, FFF—free fibula flap.

Age before Treatment y.o.	Previous Procedures	Side	Type of Flap	Number of Pieces	Soft Tissue Island	Complications	VSP and IPS	Time of Observation in Months
4		left	FFF	2	Yes	No	No	59
4		right	FFF	1	No	Bone resorption	No	77
4		right	FFF	1	Yes	No	Yes	15
5		left	FFF	2	Yes	No	Yes	9
5		left	FFF	1	Yes	No	Yes	17
5	CCG	left	FFF	2	No	No	Yes	24
5		right	FFF	2	Yes	Partial bone resorption	Yes	24
7		right	FFF	1	No	No	Yes	33
8		left	FFF	2	Yes	No	Yes	37
9		left	FFF	2	Yes	No	Yes	43
14		left	FFF	2	Yes	No	Yes	47
15		right	FFF	2	Yes	No	Yes	53
17	CCG	right	FFF	2	No	No	Yes	69

Six patients from the study group underwent DO after FFFR (Figure 3). In these patients, the bilateral DO of the mandibular body was performed. This was for increasing the advancement of the mandible. Patients eligible for DO were aged 6 (three patients), 8, 10, and 12 years. Four of these patients had tracheostomy before reconstructive treatment was started. The remaining patients had severe respiratory disorders confirmed by PSG, with high levels of AHI: above 20. In three patients, the tracheostomy was removed after FFFR. In one patient, the tracheostomy was not removed. This patient had a complication in the form of bone flap resorption; no distraction was performed. In the remaining patients, after FFFR, respiratory improvement was observed, and AHI decreased by 8 AHI units on average.

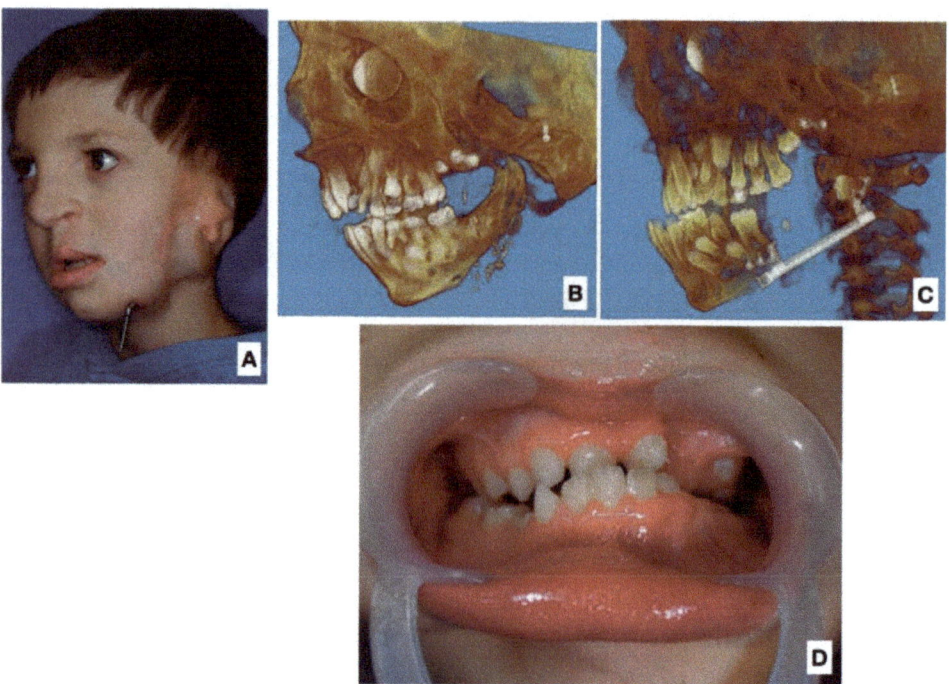

Figure 3. The same patient two years after surgery. (**A**) Three-quarter view after completion of osteodistraction. (**B**) 3D image reconstruction after FFF reconstruction. (**C**) 3D image reconstruction after completion of mandibular distraction. (**D**) Intraoral view with visible overcorrection and dentition set in reverse occlusion.

Bilateral DO of the mandibular body was performed in six patients. DO was not performed in the other seven patients because the respiratory parameters were good and there were no indications for further treatment. One patient was a teenager (aged 15 years) and FFFR combined with orthognathic surgery was sufficient to correct the defect. DO was repeated in two patients later, correcting asymmetry and malocclusion. One patient underwent DO of the mandibular ramus to prepare for FFFR. Four patients had tracheostomy before FFFR treatment. The AHI before FFFR in non-tracheostomy patients was over 20 in all cases, with a mean of 20,0. After FFFR, the tracheostomy was removed in three patients. In the remaining patients, the AHI after FFFR ranged from 12 to 21 (mean 11.4). The patient with the highest AHI, 22, was a tracheostomy patient.

During the growth of the patients, respiratory parameters deteriorated over time, reaching high AHI values. Indications for DO include exacerbating OSAS confirmed clinically and on PSG (AHI from 18 to 24, mean 21.5). The time between FFFR and DO was two years in four patients, three years in two patients, and five years in one patient. There was a two-year interval between FFFR and DO in younger children who underwent FFF reconstruction at the age of four. Subsequently, during follow-up examinations, respiratory parameters (AHI) deteriorated in 6 patients (AHI from 18 to 24, mean 21.5). These patients were qualified for mandibular DO to open the upper airways and improve breathing. The average AHI after distraction was 12 index. Improvements were noted in this context [18] (Table 3).

Table 3. Analysis of OSA based on AHI in patients undergoing FFFR, after fibular flap reconstruction. FFFR—free fibula flap reconstruction, TMR—temporo mandibular reconstruction alloplastic prosthesis, BIMAX—orthognathic bimaxillary surgery, TRACHEO—tracheostomy, DO—distraction osteogenesis, n—no tracheostomy, y—yes tracheostomy.

Age before Treatment y.o.	TRACHEO before FFFR	Tracheostomy Removal	AHI before FFFR	AHI after FFFR	AHI before DO	Age during DO y.o.	AHI after DO	Additional Surgery
4	n	n	26	16	22	6	10	
4	n	n	24	15	23	6	13	
4	y	y	TRACHEO	16	22	6	12	
5	n	n	23	11	18	8	16	
5	y	n	TRACHEO	21	24	8	12	
5	n	n	20	19	18	No DO	No DO/9	
5	y	y	TRACHEO	13	17	No DO	No DO/10	
7	y	n	TRACHEO	TRACHO	TRACHO	No DO	TRACHEO	
8	n	n	20	12	20	13	12	
9	n	n	17	10	15	No DO	No DO/9	
14	n	n	16	12	18	No DO	No DO/11	TMR/BIMAX
15	y	y	27	11	16	No DO	No DO/11	TMR/BIMAX
17	n	n	20	12	16	No DO	No DO/11	TMR/BIMAX

4. Discussion

The clinical evaluation of the patient for presumptive OSA is an essential first step in diagnosis. The assessment is based on the key symptoms of sleep apnea: snoring or witnessing a stop in breathing during sleep, insomnia, sleep hygiene, and the patient's sleep schedule. Other symptoms, such as restless legs syndrome or parasomnias, should be excluded as possible contributing factors to the patient's complaints. The physical examination for patients with suspected OSA was comprehensive and included the assessment of blood pressure, obesity index, and nose, throat, and craniofacial functions. The classification system for OSA in children is still being discussed and has not yet been standardized. Large observational studies of healthy children were conducted to define reference values for respiratory parameters during sleep [19]. Interestingly, reference values for common PSG parameters, such as AHI, do not follow a normal distribution. Tonsillectomy and adenoidectomy are the mainstay of pediatric OSA treatment. A small group of pediatric patients with OSA will still have respiratory disorders, which indicates a craniofacial etiology [20]. Continuous positive airway pressure (CPAP) is therefore indicated for treatment until surgical intervention can be performed to correct the skeletal abnormality that produces this disease. CPAP is relatively well tolerated in a large proportion of these patients, with studies reporting up to 80% adherence [21]. However, achieving good CPAP mask adherence in craniofacial pediatric patients is quite difficult. Additionally, it can be a potential limitation of CPAP in the pediatric population.

The most difficult and challenging patients are those with advanced mandibular hypoplasia causing respiratory distress and increasing asymmetry to decreasing saturation, leading to the need for tracheostomy. Many patients with mild to moderate mandibular deformities can be treated successfully with a combination of these techniques, but these procedures are often not sufficient to adequately reconstruct the severely hypoplastic mandible deformity. This makes it more challenging to treat younger patients with this type of deformity. The need for tracheostomy is still an important element affecting the patient's development. On the other hand, if early reconstruction stimulated by osteogenic DO is not performed, the asymmetry aggravates and prevents successful reconstructions at a later age. FFFR has become an invaluable tool in mandibular reconstruction, and it has a significant advantage over bone grafting and DO in complex or severe mandibular hypoplasia [18]. Non-vascularized bone grafts, such as CCG and iliac crest bone grafts, have a high percentage of atrophy and failure [22]. These grafts show high rates of resorption or unpredictable growth patterns or may lead to ankylosis [23–25]. In addition to a poorly vascularized recipient bed, these patients have hypoplastic fibrotic soft tissues on the affected side, which induces high pressure on the inserted bone graft, also affecting faster resorption. The high failure rate of the free non-vascularized grafts in CFM is a consequence of defective surrounding soft tissues. In the case of the patients in our study group, all microsurgical FFF grafts were performed initially, and in contrast to the reported cases, two cases were two patients after multiple reconstructions with CCG grafts and one teenage patient not treated previously. CCGs are a choice for the reconstruction of the mandibulae. Cartilage is the center of growth in the literature; however, this growth is unpredictable and can range from no growth to hypertrophy. CCG can be taken at the age of about 10 years due to the development of the chest, which significantly delays the possibility of reconstruction and the planning of the next stages of treatment. It can also lead to damage of the upper respiratory tract by tracheostomy. In today's era of microsurgery, it is not too aggressive to harvest a fibula from a young patient. It is no less aggressive to take CCG and wait for the chest to grow, which delays the start of the patient's respiratory rehabilitation.

DO of CCG has a high complication rate, up to 68% [26]. Complications include device failure, no healing, temporomandibular joint ankylosis, and the lack of consolidation, but DO of costochondral grafts is still possible [27]. The authors note that FFFs have a low resorption rate compared with non-vascularized bone grafts and are stable over time [28]. We no longer consider non-vascularized bone grafts to be the best option in this group of patients, and in recent cases, bone grafting was attempted before free flap surgery. It can be seen from the presented material that mandibular DO was intended to enlarge the upper airway, causing the reduction of OSAs which are destructive to children's overall development. These patients, if untreated, would probably have been condemned to tracheostomy. In the case of two patients, permanent tracheostomy could be removed after reconstruction. This demonstrates the effectiveness of the method and the disappearance of the problem of respiratory disorders associated with severe mandibular hypoplasia.

The reconstruction of the mandible in CFM using different donor flaps has been reported. Mandibular reconstruction using scapular flaps to restore facial symmetry have been reported [29]. FFF is the predominantly used flap for mandibular reconstruction in children due to the ability to collect a large amount of bone, ease of preparation, ability to collect a simultaneous soft-tissue flap for soft-tissue reconstruction, low incidence of complications at the donor site, and ability to perform effective DO [30]. Additional benefits include the ability to perform multiple osteotomies without compromising blood supply and the use of septocutaneous perforators to obtain soft tissue for facial contour reconstruction. The anatomy of FFF allows the bone to be divided into multiple segments and a double bar created to achieve adequate alveolar height and anatomical contour. The volume of good quality bone in FFF allows for the placement of dental implants or TMR prostheses, which is crucial for obtaining proper dentition (Figure 4). Early FFF grafting allows for the improvement and reconstruction of the posterior facial height and successful mandibular DO, even in a multistage protocol, to catch up with the growth disorder at a later stage. It allows for the final reconstruction with allopathic joint implants. FFF can be used successfully in patients who have undergone multiple previous surgeries in the same surgical field, including failed bone grafts and DO or previous free flaps for soft tissue augmentation. There is no objective evidence for bone flap growth. Studies show continued mandibular growth of the residual natural mandible [31]. The analysis has shown that "growth potential" was observed in 58% of patients. Factors associated with improved growth potential include condylar preservation in reconstructions performed between 8 and 12 y.o., when there is a period of rapid mandibular growth [10].

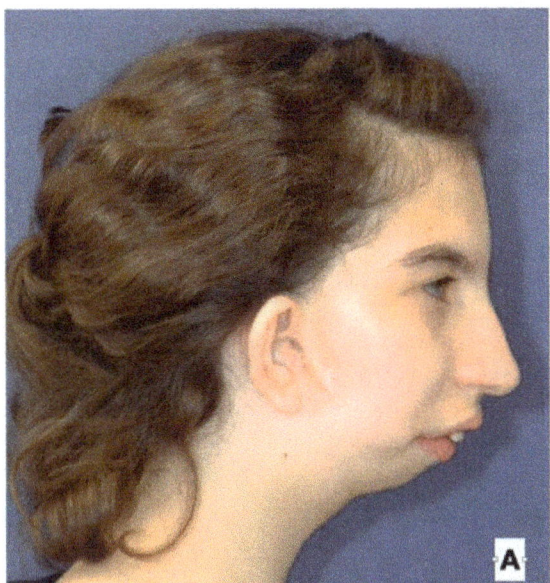 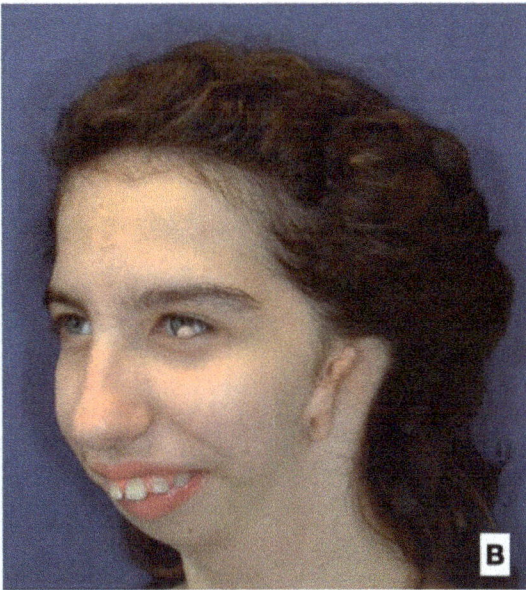

Figure 4. Patient aged 15 years with bilateral HFM. (**A**) Side view. (**B**) Three-quarter view.

The development of virtual surgical planning technology has resulted in significant advances in complex craniofacial surgery (Figure 5) [32]. Its use facilitates complex, multiplanar bone movements and allows the reconstructive surgeon to accurately predict postoperative anatomical relationships. Virtual preoperative planning also allows the precise coordination of resection and reconstruction. Prefabricated cutting instruments reduce surgery time and allow excellent bone contact between the mandibular bone fragments and the transferred bone, which contributes to better results. In the case of Pruzansky IIB, III mandibular reconstruction in patients with severe facial CFM, virtual surgical planning is particularly important. These patients have an asymmetric skull base and no mandibular fossa, making it very difficult to determine where the fibula should be located (Figure 5).

Our philosophy is that FFFR is mainly to open the upper airway. In the next step, it is used to prevent progressive asymmetry by aligning the mandibular position and rebuilding the height on the deficient side. In addition, the graft is a preparation for possible DO in the future.

In our material, mandibular DO was performed in six cases. In OSAS cases, patients warranted subsequent DO. Our cases involving DO around the age of 6 support this hypothesis. DO significantly improves the symmetry and conditions of the underlying soft tissues.

With time and follow-up, we will be better able to determine the optimal timing for performing mandibular microvascular reconstruction and subsequent DO, and finally possible alloplastic TMJ reconstruction. We can continue observing the development of patients and assessing the growth of the transplanted bone. We can monitor the assessment of the quality of life based on questionnaires and the final objective assessment of the treatment effects after reaching adulthood, based on the number of procedures performed, the number of complications, and the achieved effects of OSA reduction, and the effects of mandibular function, the possibility of orthodontic, and implant treatment, and finally aesthetic effects.

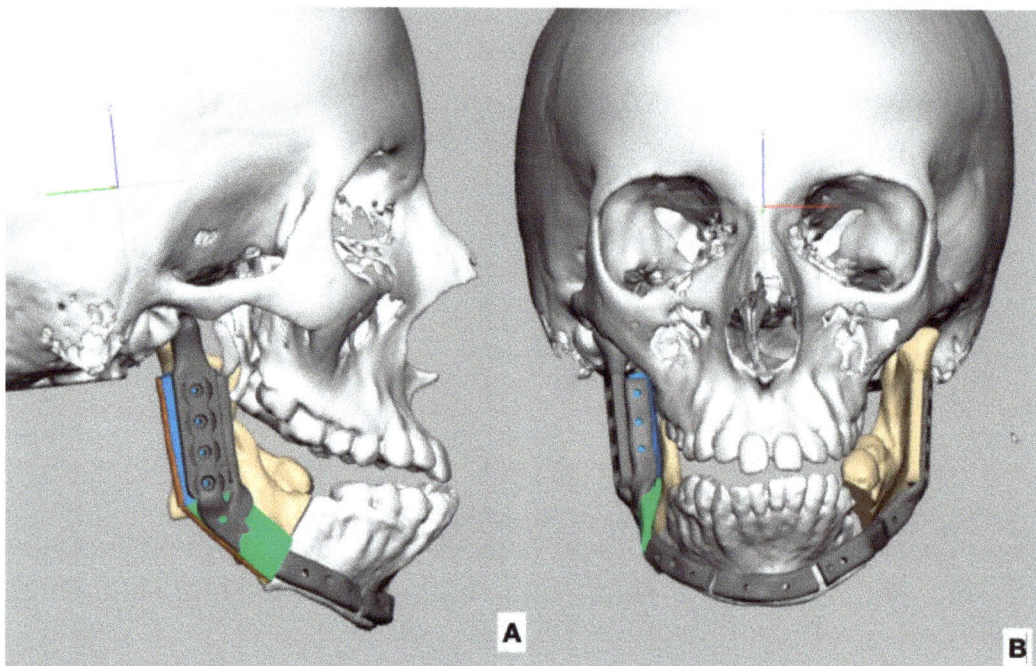

Figure 5. 3D image reconstruction. (**A**) Plan of FFF mandibular ramus reconstruction in combination with TMJ alloplastic prosthesis. (**B**) Frontal view of the plan of FFF mandibular ramus reconstruction, planned additional mandibular osteotomy on the left side.

Perhaps the main advantage of employing FFFR is the ability for reproducible DO with associated benefits. As there is no mandibular fossa, the addition of a cartilaginous fibular head would still not result in the formation of the temporomandibular joint. We did not observe FFF growth, but we did note "remodeling" of the distal flap in the temporal bone zone and resorption in two cases. The remodeling of the distal part was observed in CT scans performed 6 months after surgery and in patients qualified for DO. Remodeling consisted of smoothing the sharp bone edges and shortening the distal part. One patient developed ankylosis between the fragment and the temporal bone, which was removed during the DO procedure.

The study was performed on a small group of patients due to the rarity of this type of pathology and indications for surgical intervention. Radiation protection of growing children is a limitation for CT assessment. On the other hand, clinical and polysomnographic examinations were performed every 6 months to find indications for possible DO. Observations will continue to be carried out to assess the effects of treatment and patients' growth, especially after reaching maturity. Future areas of research include whether and by how much to overcorrect FFFR and when to perform DO. Finally, research is needed to answer the question of whether, after adequate bone aging in patients after FFFR and DO, TMJ reconstructive procedures will be needed.

5. Conclusions

The use of FFF may favorably affect the opening of the upper respiratory tract, reducing OSA. Some cases require subsequent DO. The continuous observation and assessment of apnea in this group of patients is necessary. It can be concluded that a hypoplastic mandible in CFM can be treated with good results. The FFF method, performed with virtual surgical planning, is proving to be an effective alternative to more traditional methods of mandibular reconstruction. In the cases of mandibular hypoplasia, the mandibular microvascular reconstruction with FFF can be considered a primary reconstruction modality. The FFF flap may serve as excellent material for subsequent DO, as well as bimaxillary surgery as the final stage of the treatment. FFF reconstruction with subsequent DO significantly improves respiratory function in patients with CFM.

Author Contributions: Conceptualization, K.D.; formal analysis, K.D., R.P., A.M. and Ł.K.; investigation, Ł.K.; data curation, R.P.; writing—original draft, K.D.; writing—review & editing, K.D.; supervision, A.M. All authors have read and agreed to the published version of the manuscript.

Funding: This research was funded by CHM SP. Z O.O. (Lewickie, Poland).

Institutional Review Board Statement: The Bioethics Committee for Scientific Research at the Academy of Physical Education in Katowice, No. 1/2021, 28 October 2021.

Informed Consent Statement: Informed consent was obtained from all subjects involved in the study.

Data Availability Statement: The data are available upon request from the corresponding author.

Conflicts of Interest: The authors declare no conflict of interest.

References

1. Birgfeld, C.; Heike, C. Craniofacial Microsomia. *Clin. Plast. Surg.* **2019**, *46*, 207–221. [CrossRef] [PubMed]
2. Wink, J.D.; Goldstein, J.A.; Paliga, J.T.; Taylor, J.A.; Bartlett, S.P. The mandibular deformity in hemifacial microsomia: A reassessment of the pruzansky and kaban classification. *Plast. Reconstr. Surg.* **2014**, *133*, 174–181. [CrossRef] [PubMed]
3. Heike, C.L.; Wallace, E.; Speltz, M.L.; Siebold, B.; Werler, M.M.; Hing, A.V.; Birgfeld, C.B.; Collett, B.R.; Leroux, B.G.; Luquetti, D.V. Characterizing facial features in individuals with craniofacial microsomia: A systematic approach for clinical research. *Birth Defects Res. Part A Clin. Mol. Teratol.* **2016**, *106*, 915–926. [CrossRef] [PubMed]
4. Heike, C.L.; Hing, A.V.; Aspinall, C.A.; Bartlett, S.P.; Birgfeld, C.B.; Drake, A.F.; Pimenta, L.A.; Sie, K.C.; Urata, M.M.; Vivaldi, D.; et al. Clinical care in craniofacial microsomia: A review of current management recommendations and opportunities to advance research. *Am. J. Med. Genet. Part C Semin. Med. Genet.* **2013**, *163*, 271–282. [CrossRef]
5. Padwa, B. Indications for neonatal and pediatric distraction. *Int. J. Oral Maxillofac. Surg.* **2011**, *40*, 1011. [CrossRef]
6. Brevi, B.C.; Leporati, M.; Sesenna, E. Neonatal mandibular distraction in a patient with Treacher Collins syndrome. *J. Craniofacial Surg.* **2015**, *26*, e44–e48. [CrossRef]
7. Pluijmers, B.I.; Caron, C.J.J.M.; Dunaway, D.J.; Wolvius, E.B.; Koudstaal, M.J. Mandibular reconstruction in the growing patient with unilateral craniofacial microsomia: A systematic review. *Int. J. Oral Maxillofac. Surg.* **2014**, *43*, 286–295. [CrossRef]
8. Hidalgo, D.A. Fibula free flap: A new method of mandible reconstruction. *Plast. Reconstr. Surg.* **1989**, *84*, 71–79. [CrossRef]
9. Aboelatta, Y.A.; Aly, H.M. Free Tissue Transfer and Replantation in Pediatric Patients: Technical Feasibility and Outcome in a Series of 28 Patients. *J. Hand Microsurg.* **2016**, *5*, 74–80. [CrossRef]
10. Temiz, G.; Bilkay, U.; Tiftikçioğlu, Y.Ö.; Mezili, C.T.; Songür, E. The evaluation of flap growth and long-term results of pediatric mandible reconstructions using free fibular flaps. *Microsurgery* **2015**, *35*, 253–261. [CrossRef]
11. Cleveland, E.C.; Zampell, J.; Avraham, T.; Lee, Z.-H.; Hirsch, D.; Levine, J.P. Reconstruction of congenital mandibular hypoplasia with microvascular free fibula flaps in the pediatric population: A paradigm shift. *J. Craniofacial Surg.* **2017**, *28*, 79–83. [CrossRef] [PubMed]
12. Caron, C.; Pluijmers, B.; Maas, B.; Klazen, Y.; Katz, E.; Abel, F.; van der Schroeff, M.; Mathijssen, I.; Dunaway, D.; Mills, C.; et al. Obstructive sleep apnoea in craniofacial microsomia: Analysis of 755 patients. *Int. J. Oral Maxillofac. Surg.* **2017**, *46*, 1330–1337. [CrossRef] [PubMed]
13. Wei, F.-C.; Demirkan, F.; Chen, H.-C.; Chen, I.-H. Double free flaps in reconstruction of extensive composite mandibular defects in head and neck cancer. *Plast. Reconstr. Surg.* **1999**, *103*, 39–47. [CrossRef] [PubMed]
14. Scott, A.R.; Tibesar, R.J.; Sidman, J.D. Pierre Robin Sequence. Evaluation, Management, Indications for Surgery, and Pitfalls. *Otolaryngol. Clin. N. Am.* **2012**, *45*, 695–710. [CrossRef] [PubMed]
15. Cielo, C.M.; Marcus, C.L. Obstructive sleep apnoea in children with craniofacial syndromes. *Paediatr. Respir. Rev.* **2015**, *16*, 189–196. [CrossRef]
16. Katz, E.S.; D'Ambrosio, C.M. Pediatric obstructive sleep apnea syndrome. *Clin. Chest Med.* **2010**, *31*, 221–234. [CrossRef]
17. Marcus, C.L.; Brooks, L.J.; Draper, K.A.; Gozal, D.; Halbower, A.C.; Jones, J.; Schechter, M.S.; Sheldon, S.H.; Spruyt, K.; Ward, S.D.; et al. Diagnosis and management of childhood obstructive sleep apnea syndrome. *Pediatrics* **2012**, *130*, 576–584. [CrossRef]
18. Damlar, İ.; Altan, A.; Turgay, B.; Kiliç, S. Management of obstructive sleep apnea in a Treacher Collins syndrome patient using distraction osteogenesis of the mandible. *J. Korean Assoc. Oral Maxillofac. Surg.* **2016**, *42*, 388. [CrossRef]
19. Uliel, S.; Tauman, R.; Greenfeld, M.; Sivan, Y. Normal polysomnographic respiratory values in children and adolescents. *Chest* **2004**, *125*, 872–878. [CrossRef]

20. Lin, S.-Y.; Su, Y.-X.; Wu, Y.-C.; Chang, J.Z.-C.; Tu, Y.-K. Management of paediatric obstructive sleep apnoea: A systematic review and network meta-analysis. *Int. J. Paediatr. Dent.* **2020**, *30*, 156–170. [CrossRef]
21. Marcus, C.L.; Ward, S.L.D.; Mallory, G.B.; Rosen, C.L.; Beckerman, R.C.; Weese-Mayer, D.E.; Brouillette, R.T.; Trang, H.T.; Brooks, L.J. Use of nasal continuous positive airway pressure as treatment of childhood obstructive sleep apnea. *J. Pediatr.* **1995**, *127*, 88–94. [CrossRef] [PubMed]
22. Tahiri, Y.; Chang, C.S.; Tuin, J.; Paliga, J.T.; Lowe, K.M.; Taylor, J.A.; Bartlett, S.P. Costochondral grafting in craniofacial microsomia. *Plast. Reconstr. Surg.* **2015**, *135*, 530–541. [CrossRef] [PubMed]
23. Fernandes, R.; Fattahi, T.; Steinberg, B. Costochondral Rib Grafts in Mandibular Reconstruction. *Atlas Oral Maxillofac. Surg. Clin.* **2006**, *14*, 179–183. [CrossRef] [PubMed]
24. Merkx, M.A.W.; Freihofer, H.P.M. Fracture of costochondral graft in temporomandibular joint reconstructive surgery: An unexpected complication. *Int. J. Oral Maxillofac. Surg.* **1995**, *24*, 142–144. [CrossRef] [PubMed]
25. Yang, S.; Fan, H.; Du, W.; Li, J.; Hu, J.; Luo, E. Overgrowth of costochondral grafts in craniomaxillofacial reconstruction: Rare complication and literature review. *J. Cranio-Maxillofac. Surg.* **2015**, *43*, 803–812. [CrossRef]
26. Chan, C.; Włodarczyk, J.R.; Wolfswinkel, E.M.; Odono, L.T.; Urata, M.M.; Hammoudeh, J.A. Establishing a Novel Treatment Algorithm for Pediatric Mandibular Tumor Reconstruction. *J. Craniofacial Surg.* **2022**, *33*, 744–749. [CrossRef]
27. Acosta, H.L.; Stelnicki, E.J.; Boyd, J.B.; Barnavon, Y.; Uecker, C. Vertical mesenchymal distraction and bilateral free fibula transfer for severe Treacher Collins syndrome. *Plast. Reconstr. Surg.* **2004**, *113*, 1209–1217. [CrossRef]
28. Shokri, T.; Stahl Bs, L.E.; Kanekar, S.G.; Goyal, N. Osseous Changes Over Time in Free Fibular Flap Reconstruction. *Laryngoscope* **2019**, *129*, 1113–1116. [CrossRef]
29. Warren, S.M.; Borud, L.J.; Brecht, L.E.; Longaker, M.T.; Siebert, J.W. Microvascular reconstruction of the pediatric mandible. *Plast. Reconstr. Surg.* **2007**, *119*, 649–661. [CrossRef]
30. Dowgierd, K.; Pokrowiecki, R.; Borowiec, M.; Kozakiewicz, M.; Smyczek, D.; Krakowczyk, Ł. A protocol for the use of a combined microvascular free flap with custom-made 3d-printed total temporomandibular joint (TMJ) prosthesis for mandible reconstruction in children. *Appl. Sci.* **2021**, *11*, 2176. [CrossRef]
31. Zhang, W.-B.; Liang, T.; Peng, X. Mandibular growth after paediatric mandibular reconstruction with the vascularized free fibula flap: A systematic review. *Int. J. Oral Maxillofac. Surg.* **2016**, *45*, 440–447. [CrossRef] [PubMed]
32. Krakowczyk, Ł.; Piotrowska-Seweryn, A.; Szymczyk, C.; Wierzgoń, J.; Oleś, K.; Ulczok, R.; Donocik, K.; Dowgierd, K.; Maciejewski, A. Virtual surgical planning and cone beam computed tomography in reconstruction of head and neck tumors—Pilot study. *Otolaryngol. Pol.* **2020**, *74*, 28–33. [CrossRef] [PubMed]

Disclaimer/Publisher's Note: The statements, opinions and data contained in all publications are solely those of the individual author(s) and contributor(s) and not of MDPI and/or the editor(s). MDPI and/or the editor(s) disclaim responsibility for any injury to people or property resulting from any ideas, methods, instructions or products referred to in the content.

MDPI
St. Alban-Anlage 66
4052 Basel
Switzerland
www.mdpi.com

Journal of Clinical Medicine Editorial Office
E-mail: jcm@mdpi.com
www.mdpi.com/journal/jcm

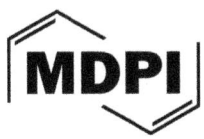

Disclaimer/Publisher's Note: The statements, opinions and data contained in all publications are solely those of the individual author(s) and contributor(s) and not of MDPI and/or the editor(s). MDPI and/or the editor(s) disclaim responsibility for any injury to people or property resulting from any ideas, methods, instructions or products referred to in the content.

www.ingramcontent.com/pod-product-compliance
Lightning Source LLC
LaVergne TN
LVHW070554100526
838202LV00012B/464